高等教育出版社 中国·北京
Higher Education Press, Beijing, China

英漢實用中醫藥大全

趙樸初題

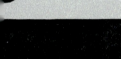

醫學氣功

THE ENGLISH-CHINESE ENCYCLOPEDIA OF PRACTICAL TRDITIONAL CHINESE MEDICINE

Chief Editor	Xu Xiangcai	
Assistants	You Ke	Kang Kai
	Bao Xuequan	Lu Yubin

英汉实用中医药大全

主　编	徐象才	
主编助理	尤　可	康　凯
	鲍学全	路玉滨

Higher Education Press
高等教育出版社

THE ENGLISH-CHINESE ENCYCLOPEDIA OF PRACTICAL TRADITIONAL CHINESE MEDICINE

Chief Editor: Xu Xiangcai
Assistants: You Ke, Zang Ke
 Bao Zaiqun, Di Xiufen

英汉实用中医药大全

Higher Education Press
高等教育出版社

8

医 学 气 功

	中文	英文
主编	毕永升	于文平
编者	张铭琴	孙希刚
	毕珂	
审校		黄孝楷

MEDICAL *QIGONG*

	English	Chinese
Chief Editor	Yu Wenping	Bi Yongsheng
Editors	Sun Xigang	Zhang Mingqin
		Bi Ke
Reviser	Huang XiaoKai	

The Leading Commission of Compilation and Translation
编译领导委员会

Honorary Director 名誉主任委员	Hu Ximing 胡熙明			
Honorary Deputy Director 名誉副主任委员	Zhang Qiwen 张奇文	Wang Lei 王镭		
Director 主任委员	Zou Jilong 邹积隆			
Deputy Director 副主任委员	Wei Jiwu 隗继武			
Members 委员 (以姓名笔划为序)	Wan Deguang, 万德光 Cong Chunyu, 丛春雨 Qiu Dewen, 邱德文 Gao Jinliang, 高金亮 Zhai Weimin, 瞿维敏	Wang Yongyan, 王永炎 Liu Zhongben, 刘中本 Shang Chichang, 尚炽昌 Cheng Yichun, 程益春	Wang Maoze, 王懋泽 Sun Guojie, 孙国杰 Xiang Ping, 项平 Ge Linyi, 葛琳仪	Wei Guikang, 韦贵康 Yan Shiyun, 严世芸 Zhao Yisen, 赵以森 Cai Jianqian, 蔡剑前
Advisers 顾问	Dong Jianhua, 董建华 Zhou Ciqing, 周次清	Huang Xiaokai, 黄孝楷 Chen Keji, 陈可冀	Geng Jianting, 耿鉴庭	Zhou Fengwu, 周凤梧

The Commission of Compilation and Translation
编译委员会

Director　　Xu Xiangcai,
主任委员　　徐象才

Deputy Directors　Zhang Zhigang,　Zhang Wengao,　Jiang Zhaojun,　Qi Xiuheng,
副主任委员　　张志刚　　　　张文高　　　　姜兆俊　　　　亓秀恒

　　　　　　　Xuan Jiasheng,　Sun xiangxie,
　　　　　　　宣家声　　　　孙祥燮

Members　　Yu Wenping,　　Wang Zhengzhong,　Wang Chenying,　Wang Guocai,
委员　　　　　于文平　　　　王正忠　　　　　王陈应　　　　王国才
(以姓名笔划为序) Fang Tingyu,　Fang Xuwu,　　Tian Jingzhen,　Bi Yongsheng,
　　　　　　　方廷钰　　　　方续武　　　　田景振　　　　毕永升

　　　　　　　Liu Yutan,　　　Liu Chengcai,　Liu Jiaqi,　　Liu Xiaojuan,
　　　　　　　刘玉檀　　　　刘承才　　　　刘家起　　　　刘晓娟

　　　　　　　Zhu Zhongbao,　Zhu Zhenduo,　Xun Jianying,　Li Lei,
　　　　　　　朱忠宝　　　　朱振铎　　　　寻建英　　　　李磊

　　　　　　　Li Zhulan,　　Xin Shoupu,　　Shao Nianfang,　Chen Shaomin,
　　　　　　　李竹兰　　　　辛守璞　　　　邵念方　　　　陈绍民

　　　　　　　Zou Jilong,　　Lu Shengnian,　Zhou Xing,　　Zhou Ciqing,
　　　　　　　邹积隆　　　　陆胜年　　　　周行　　　　　周次清

　　　　　　　Zhang Sufang,　Yang Chongfeng,　Zhao Chunxiu,　Yu Changzheng,
　　　　　　　张素芳　　　　杨崇峰　　　　赵纯修　　　　俞昌正

　　　　　　　Hu Zunda,　　Xu Heying,　　Yuan Jiurong,　Huang Naijian,
　　　　　　　胡遵达　　　　须鹤瑛　　　　袁久荣　　　　黄乃健

　　　　　　　Huang Kuiming,　Huang Jialing,　Cao Yixun,　　Lei Xilian,
　　　　　　　黄奎铭　　　　黄嘉陵　　　　曹贻训　　　　雷希濂

　　　　　　　Cai Huasong,　Cai Jianqian,
　　　　　　　蔡华松　　　　蔡剑前

Preface

I am delighted to learn that THE ENGLISH—CHINESE ENCYCLOPEDIA OF PRACTICAL TRADITIONAL CHINESE MEDICINE will soon come into the world.

TCM has experienced many vicissitudes of times but has remained evergreen. It has made great contributions not only to the power and prosperity of our Chinese nation but to the enrichment and improvement of world medicine. Unfortunately, differences in nations, states and languages have slowed down its spreading and flowing outside China. At present, however, an upsurge in learning, researching and applying TCM is unfolding. In order to maximize the effect of this upsurge and to lead TCM, one of the brilliant cultural heritages of the Chinese nation, to the world for it to expand and bring benefit to the people of all nations, Mr.Xu Xiangcai called intellectuals of noble aspirations and high intelligence together from Shandong and many other provinces in China. and took charge of the work of both compilation and translation of THE ENGLISH—CHINESE ENCYCLOPEDIA OF PRACTICAL TRADITIONAL CHINESE MEDICINE. With great pleasure, the medical staff both at home and abroad will hail the appearance of this encyclopedia.

I believe that the day when the world's medicine is fully developed will be the day when TCM has spread throughout the world.

I have written my preface with pleasure.

By Prof. Dr. Hu Ximing

> Deputy minister of the Ministry of Public Health of the People's Republic of China,
>
> Director general of The State Administrative Bureau of Traditional Chinese Medicine and Pharmacology,
>
> President of The World Federation of Acupuncture-Moxibustion Societies,
>
> Member of China Association of Science & Technology,
>
> Deputy president of All-China Association of Traditional Chinese Medicine.
>
> President of China Acupuncture & Moxibustion Society.

December, 1989.

Preface

The Chinese Nation has been through a long, arduous course of struggling against diseases and has developed its own traditional medicine—Traditional Chinese Medicine and Pharmacology (TCMP). TCMP has a unique, comprehensive, scientific system including both theories and clinical practice. Some thousand years since its beginnings, not only has it been well preserved but also continuously developed. It has special advan tages, such as remarkable curative effects and few side effects. Hence it is an effective means by which people prevent and treat diseases and keep themselves strong and healthy.

All achievements attained by any nation in the development of medicine are the public wealth of all mankind. They should not be confined within a single country. What is more, the need to set them free to flow throughout the world as quickly and precisely as possible is greater than that of any other kind of science. During my more than thirty years of being engaged in Traditional Chinese Medicine (TCM), I have been looking forward to the day when TCMP will have spread all over the world and made its contributions to the elimination of diseases of all mankind. However it is to be deeply regretted that the pace of TCMP in extending outside China has been unsatisfactory due to the major difficulties in expressing its concepts and methods in foreign languages.

Mr.Xu Xiangcai, a teacher of Shandong College of TCM,

has sponsored and taken charge of the work of compilation and translation of The English—Chinese Encyclopedia of Practical Traditional Chinese Medicine —an extensive series. This work is a great project, a large—scale scientific research, a courageous effort and a novel creation. I deeply esteem Mr. Xu Xiangcai and his compilers and translators for their hard labor, working day and night for such a long time, for their firm and indomitable will displayed in overcoming one difficulty after another, and for their great success achieved in this way. As a leader in the circles of TCM, I am duty—bound to try my best to support them.

I believe this encyclopedia will be certain to find its position both in the history of Chinese medicine and in the history of world science and technology.

By Mr. Zhang Qiwen
Member of The Standing Committee of
All—China Association of TCM,
Deputy head of The Health Department of
Shandong Province.
March , 1990.

Publisher's Preface

Traditional Chinese Medicine (TCM) is one of China's great cultural heritages. Since the founding of the People's Republic of China in 1949, guided by the farsighted TCM policy of the Chinese Communist Party and the Chinese government, the treasure house of the theories of TCM has been continuously explored and the plentiful literature researched and compiled. As a result, great success has been achieved. Today there has appeared a world-wide upsurge in the studying and researching of TCM. To promote even more vigorous development of this trend in order that TCM may better serve all mankind, efforts are required to further it throughout the world. To bring this about, the language barriers must be overcome as soon as possible in order that TCM can be accurately expressed in foreign languages.

Thus the compilation and translation of a series of Chinese-English books of basic knowledge of TCM has become of great urgency to serve the needs of medical and educational circles both inside and outside China.

In recent years, at the request of the health departments, satisfactory achievements have been made in researching the expression of TCM in English. Based on the investigation into the history and current state of the research work mentioned above, The English-Chinese Encyclopedia of Practical TCM has been published to meet the needs of extending the knowledge of TCM around the world.

The encyclopedia consists of twenty-one volumes, each dealing with a particular branch of TCM. In the process of compilation, the distinguishing features of TCM have been given close attention and great efforts have been made to ensure that the content is scientific, practical, comprehensive and concise. The chief writers of the Chinese manuscripts include professors or associate professors with at least twenty years of practical clinical and / or teaching experience in TCM. The Chinese manuscript of each volume has been checked and approved by a specialist of the relevant branch of TCM. The team of the translators and revisers of the English versions consists of TCM specialists with a good command of English, professional medical translators, and teachers of English from TCM colleges or universities, At a symposium to standardize the English versions, scholars from twenty-two colleges or universities, research institutes of TCM or other health institutes probed the questions of how to express TCM in English more comprehensively, systematically and accurately, and discussed and deliberated in detail the English versions of some volumes inorder to upgrade the English versions of the whole series. The English version of each volume has been re-examined and then given a final checking.

Obviously this encyclopedia will provide extensive reading material of TCM English for senior students in colleges of TCM in China and will also greatly benefit foreigners studying TCM.

The assiduous efforts of compiling and translating this encyclopedia have been supported by the responsible leaders of the State Education Commission of the People's Republic of China, the State Administrative Bureau of TCM and Pharmacy, the Education Commission and Health Department of Shandong Province.

Under the direction of the Higher Education Department of the State Education Commission, the leading board of compilation and translation of this encyclopedia was set up. The leaders of many colleges of TCM and pharmaceutical factories of TCM have also given assistance.

We hope that this encyclopedia will bring about a good effect on enhancing the teaching of TCM English at the colleges of TCM in China, on cultivating skills in medical circles in exchanging ideas of TCM with patients in English, and on giving an impetus to the study of TCM outside China.

Higher Education Press
March, 1990.

Foreword

The English—Chinese Encyclopedia of Practical Traditional Chinese Medicine is an extensive series of twenty—one volumes, Based on the fundamental theories of Traditional Chinese Medicine (TCM) and with emphasis on the clinical practice of TCM, it is a semi—advanced English—Chinese academic works which is quite comprehensive, systematic, concise, practical and easy to read. It caters mainly to the following readers: senior students of colleges of TCM, young and middle—aged teachers of colleges of TCM, young and middle—aged physicians of hospitals of TCM. personnel of scientific research institutions of TCM, teachers giving correspondence courses in TCM to foreigners, TCM personnel going abroad in the capacity of lecturers or physicians, those trained in western medicine but wishing to study TCM, and foreigners coming to China to learn TCM or to take refresher courses in TCM.

Because Traditional Chinese Medicine and Pharmacology is unique to our Chinese nation, putting TCM into English has been the crux of the compilation and translation of this encyclopedia. Owing to the fact that no one can be proficient both in the theories of Traditional Chinese Medicine and Pharmacology and the clinical practice of every branch of TCM, as well as in English, to ensure that the English versions express accurately the inherent meanings of TCM, collective translation measures have been taken. That is , teachers of English familiar with TCM, professional medical translators, teachers or physicians of TCM and even teachers of palaeography with a strong command of English were all invited together to co-translate the Chinese manuscripts and then, to co-deliberate and discuss the English versions. At last, English-speaking foreigners studying TCM or teaching English in China were asked to polish the English versions. In this way, the skills of the above translators and foreigners were merged to ensure the quality of the English versions. However, even using this method, the uncertainty that the English versions will be wholly accepted still remains. As for the Chinese manuscripts, they do reflect the essence, and give a general picture, of Traditional Chinese Medicine and Pharmacology. It is not asserted, though, that they are perfect. I whole-heartedly look forward to any criticisms or opinions from readers in order to make improvements to future editions.

More than 200 people have taken part in the activities of compiling, translating and revising this encyclopedia. They come from twenty-eight institutions in all parts of China. Among these institutions, there are fifteen colleges of TCM:Shandong, Beijing, Shanghai, Tianjin, Nanjing, Zhejiang, Anhui, Henan, Hubei, Guangxi, Guiyang, Gansu, Chengdu, Shanxi and Changchun, and scientific research centers of TCM such as China Academy of TCM and Shandong Scientific Research Institute of TCM.

The Education Commission of Shandong Province has included the compilation and translation of this encyclopedia in its scientific research projects and allocated funds accordingly. The Health Department of Shandong Province has also given financial aid together with a number of pharmaceutical factories of TCM. The subsidization from Jinan Pharmaceutical Factory of

TCM provided the impetus for the work of compilation and translation to get under way.

The success of compiling and translating this encyclopedia is not only the fruit of the collective labor of all the compilers, translators and revisers but also the result of the support of the responsible leaders of the relevant leading institutions. As the encyclopedia is going to be published. I express my heartfelt thanks to all the compilers, translators and revisers and pharmaceutical factories of TCM for their sincere cooperation, and to the specialists, professors, leaders at all levels for their warm support.

It is my most profound wish that the publication of this encyclopedia will take its role in cultivating talented persons of TCM having a very good command of TCM English and in extending, rapidly, comprehensive knowledge of TCM to all corners of the globe.

Xu Xiangcai,
Shandong College of TCM,
March, 1990.

Contents

Notes ··· 1
1 An Introduction to Medical Qigong ································· 1
  1.1 Concept and Characteristics ································· 1
  1.2 The Development of *Qigong* ································· 3
  1.3 Basic Principles of *Qigong* Exercise ······················· 10
    1.3.1 Being Both Dynamic and Static ·························· 10
    1.3.2 Being Relaxed and Static Naturally ····················· 11
    1.3.3 Coordinating the Will and *Qi* (Vital Energy) ·········· 11
    1.3.4 Combining Active Exercise with Inner Health Cultivation ·· 13
    1.3.5 Proceeding in an Orderly Way and Step by Step ·········· 13
2 Three Kinds of Regulations in Qigong ····························· 15
  2.1 Regulation of the Body (Adjustment of Posture) ·············· 15
    2.1.1 Sitting Posture ·· 15
    2.1.2 Lying Posture ·· 16
    2.1.3 Standing Posture ······································· 18
    2.1.4 Essentials of Posturization ···························· 19
  2.2 Regulation of Breathing ····································· 22
    2.2.1 Natural Respiration ···································· 22
    2.2.2 Orthodromic Abdominal Respiration ······················ 23
    2.2.3 Antidromic Abdominal Respiration ······················· 23
    2.2.4 Other Breathing Methods ································ 24
    2.2.5 Essentials of Respiration Training ····················· 24
  2.3 Regulation of Mental Activities ····························· 25

2.4 Common Points ·· 27
2.5 Points for Attention in *Qigong* Exercise ····················· 31
3 Various Qigong Exercises ·· 34
  3.1 Psychosomatic Relaxation Exercise ··························· 34
  3.2 Inner Health Cultivation Exercise ····························· 37
  3.3 Health Promotion Exercise ······································· 39
  3.4 Head—Face Exercise ··· 40
  3.5 Eye Exercise ·· 44
  3.6 Nose—Teeth Exercise ·· 47
  3.7 Ear Exercise ·· 49
  3.8 Neck Exercise ·· 50
  3.9 Shoulder—Arm Exercise ·· 53
  3.10 Chest—Hypochondrium Exercise ···························· 56
  3.11 Abdominal Exercise ·· 58
  3.12 Waist Exercise ··· 60
  3.13 Exercise of the Lower Limbs ································· 61
  3.14 Heart Regulation Exercise ····································· 63
  3.15 Spleen Regulation Exercise ···································· 68
  3.16 Lung Regulation Exercise ······································ 71
  3.17 Liver Regulation Exercise ····································· 74
  3.18 Kidney Regulation Exercise ··································· 78
  3.19 Automatic *Qi* Circulation Exercise ························ 81
  3.20 *Qi* Circulation Exercise ·· 83
  3.21 Exercise for Soothing the Liver and Improving
      Acuity of Vision ·· 85
  3.22 Exercise for Nourishing the Kidney for
      Rejuvenation ··· 90
  3.23 Exercise of Taking Essence from the Sun
      and the Moon ··· 93

3.24 *Yang*—Recuperation Exercise (*Daoyang Gong*) 95
3.25 Vital Essence Recovering Exercise 98
3.26 Filth—Elimination Exercise 100
3.27 Iron Crotch Exercise (*Tiedang Gong*) 101
3.28 *Daoyin* Exercise for Ascending and Descending *Yin* and *Yang* 111
3.29 *Daoyin* Exercise for Dredging *Ren* and *Du* Channels 113
3.30 Brocade Exercise in Six Forms (*Liuduan Jin*) 117
3.31 Nine—Turn Exercise for Longevity 122
3.32 Twelve—Form Sinew—Transforming Exercise (*Yijin Jing*) 124

4 Emitting Out—going *Qi* (*Waiqi*) 143
4.1 Training of *Qi* 143
  4.1.1 Static Exercise for Training *Qi* 143
  4.1.2 Dynamic Exercise for Training *Qi* 147
4.2 The Guiding of *Qi* 162
  4.2.1 Standing Vibrating with Palms Closed to Guide *Qi* 163
  4.2.2 Single—finger Meditation to Guide *Qi* 164
  4.2.3 Palm—pushing and Palm—pulling to Guide *Qi* 165
  4.2.4 Making Three Points Linear to Guide *Qi* ... 166
  4.2.5 Making Three Points Circular to Guide *Qi* .. 167
  4.2.6 Jumping to Guide *Qi* in Burst 168
  4.2.7 Guiding *Qi* in Fixed Form 169
  4.2.8 Guiding *Qi* in Spiralty 170
  4.2.9 Cold and Heat Guidance of *Qi* 171
4.3 Emission of *Qi* 172

  4.3.1 Hand Gestures for Emitting *Qi* ·················· 172
  4.3.2 Hand Manipulations in Emitting *Qi* ············· 174
  4.3.3 The Forms of *Qi* on Emission ················· 178
  4.3.4 The Sensation of *Qi* ·························· 180
  4.3.5 The Effect of *Qi* ···························· 182
  4.3.6 The Closing Form of Emission of *Qi* ············ 184

5 Treatment ·· 185
 5.1 Deviation of *Qigong* ····································· 185
  5.1.1 Deranged Flow of *Qi* ·························· 186
  5.1.2 Stagnation of *Qi* and Stasis of Blood ············· 187
  5.1.3 Leaking of Genuine *Qi* (Vital *Qi*) ·············· 189
  5.1.4 Mental Derangement ····························· 190
  5.1.5 Management of Temporary Symptoms Emerging during
    Qigong Exercise ································ 192
 5.2 Syncope ··· 194
 5.3 Common Cold ··· 196
 5.4 Epigastralgia ··· 197
 5.5 Appendicitis ··· 200
 5.6 Disorders of the Biliary Tract ······························ 202
 5.7 Hiccup ··· 204
 5.8 Gastroptosia ··· 205
 5.9 Diarrhoea ··· 207
 5.10 Constipation ·· 209
 5.11 Hypochondriac Pain ······································ 212
 5.12 Bronchitis ·· 213
 5.13 Bronchial Asthma ······································· 216
 5.14 Palpitation ··· 218
 5.15 Seminal Emission ······································· 220
 5.16 Impotence ··· 221

5.17 Dysmenorrhea ································ 223
5.18 Chronic Pelvic Inflammation ················ 224
5.19 Metroptosis ··································· 226
5.20 Acute Mastitis ································ 228
5.21 Stiff-neck ····································· 229
5.22 Pain in the Waist and Lower Extremities ············ 230
5.23 Headache ····································· 232
5.24 Insomnia ····································· 235
5.25 Hypertension ································ 238
5.26 Cervical Spondylopathy ····················· 240
5.27 Hemiplegia ·································· 242
5.28 Myopia ······································· 243
5.29 Infantile Convulsion ························· 244
5.30 Infantile Diarrhoea ··························· 245

Notes

"Medical *Qigong*" is the eighth volume of "The English-Chinese Encyclopaedia of Practical Traditional Chinese Medicine".

This volume falls into two categories: self-controlled *Qigong* autotherapy and out-*going-Qi* therapy. The former refers to *Qigong* exercises done by patients themselves to keep fit or to cure their own illness, while the latter is the skill of *Qigong* masters to treat patients by emitting *Qi*.

The volume consists of five parts: An Introduction to Medical *Qigong*, The Three Kinds of Regulation of *Qigong*, Various *Qigong* Exercises, Emission of Out-going *Qi*, and Treatment. While presenting briefly the basic knowledge of *Qigong*, the volume gives emphasis on the skills for self-controlled autotherapy and techniques of training *Qi*, guiding *Qi* and emitting out-going *Qi*.

Treatment is the clinical application of *Qigong*. Apart from the introduction to the aetiology, pathology and symptoms of diseases, the skill of self-controlled treatment and treatment by out-going *Qi* are presented in detail in the light of the principle of diffrential diagnosis and treatment.

The book is written for medical workers and *Qigong* fans in and outside China both for classroom and reference use. It is also intended for patients who practise self-controlled *Qigong* as a guide and a helper.

Acknowledgement is made to Professor Shao Guanyong, director of the Department of Medical Papaeography of

Shandong College of Traditional Chinese Medicine, for his valuable help in preparing the Chinese manuscript of the volume.

Editor

1 An Introduction to Medical *Qigong*

1.1 Concept and Characteristics

As one of the outstanding cultural legacies of the Chinese nation, *Qigong* is a kind of psychosomatic regime aimed at disease prevention and treatment, health preservation and longevity through training of mind, breathing and posture, and regulation of the physiological status of the organism. Another great virtue ascribed to *Qigong* is known as out–going–*Qi* therapy, referring to a method adopted by skilled *Qigong* practitioners to treat patients by emitting out–going *Qi*.

Qigong is the skill to train *Qi*; *Qi* here of refers to genuine *Qi* (vital energy) in the body, intrinsic *Qi* as it is otherwise called. Traditional Chinese medicine (TCM) holds that genuine *Qi* is the dynamic force of all vital functions of the human body, the training of *Qi* termed in *Qi*gong is therefore the training of the genuine *Qi*. *Daoyin*, which is also called "*Daoyin* massage" in TCM, is a special system of exercise in *Qigong* designed for health preservation or for prevention and treatment of a certain disease, a comprehensive exercise generally performed through adjustment of the body posture, regulation of breathing and mind concentration in combination with selfmassage. Another definition of *Daoyin* refers to the skill in guiding *Qi* to flow in a certain direction controlled by the mind. This can be performed only by those who have a certain background in training *Qi* and who can feel the flow of *Qi* inside the body. For instance, Inner Health Cultivation Exercise (*Neiyang Gong*), Health Promotion Exercise (*Qiangzhuang Gong*), *Qi*—nourishing Exercise (*Yangqi Gong*) and *Qi* Circulation Exercise (*Zhoutian Gong*) are *Qigong* methods with stresses laid on training intrinsic *Qi* (genuine *Qi*), while Iron Crotch Exercise (*Tiedang Gong*), Regional *Daoyin* Exercise (*Buwei Daoyin Gong*), Five—viscera Regulation Exercise (*Li Wuzang Gong*) and others, usually performed together with selfmassage, are strongly aimed at treatment of certain diseases.

One of the characteristics of *Qigong* is its speciality in use, that is, a particular form of exercise should be chosen to meet the need of a concrete condition. When a *Qigong* method is selected, two aspects must be taken into consideration —— the general improvement of the body functions as a whole and the treatment of an illness in particular. "Static" *Qigong*, aimed at training and accumulating *Qi* to build up the constitution and obtain longevity, requires ease of the posture, mind and internal organs, regulation of breathing, guarding against distracting thoughts and concentrating the mind on *Dantian* or on a certain locality of the body. But for the invalid, it is desirable to take up an exercise optimal to the treatment of the disease. For example, for those having symptoms such as palpitation and shortness of breath due to insufficiency of the heart—*Qi*, Iron Crotch Exercise (*Tiedang Gong*) may be practised to achieve rapid therapeutic effects. The selection and practice of *Qigong* according to the constitution of individuals and the nature of their illnesses in terms of cold, heat, deficiency or excess is called Differential Diagnosis and Treatment in TCM.

Another characteristic of *Qigong* is its emphasis on self health refining, as observed by the ancient Chinese that "Running water never turns stale and a door-hinge never gets worm-eaten". "*Daoyin · Anqiao*", as put forward in *Huang Di Nei Jing* (The Yellow Emperor's Canon of Internal Medicine), consists mainly of self-controlled movements of the extremities and selfmassage to guide *Qi* and blood circulation to build up the constitution and control diseases. This exercise is, to a great extent, superior to the passive methods of massage, acupuncture, drug medication and other therapies in its merits in mobilizing the vital energy and potentials of the body to prevent and cure diseases.

Simplicity and feasibility are other advantages of *Qigong*. It can be mastered simply by reading books with illustrations, with rapid and satisfactory results.

1.2 The Development of *Qigong*

Qigong, as an art of healing and health preservation, has had a long history. It has been said that people came to know treatment of diseases by "dancing" as early as four thousand years ago in the *Tang Yao* Times. Recorded in *Lu Shi Chun Qiu*(Lu's Spring and Autumn Annals or Lu's History) is that "In the beginning of *Taotang* Tribes, the sun was often shut off by heavy clouds and it rained all the time; turbulent waters overflowed their banks. People lived a gloomy and dull life, suffering rigidity of joints. Dancing was thus recommended as a remedy". From the experience of their long-term struggle with nature, the antients gradually realized that body movements, various ways of breathing and exclamations could help readjust some functions of the human body, e.g., imitating animal movements such as climbing, looking about, leaping and flying could promote vital flow of *Qi*; pronuncing "*Hi*" could decrease or increase strength, "*Ha*" could disperse heat, "*Xu*" could allay pain, and in this way, the ancient primitive *Qigong* was brought into being.

During the Spring and Autumn and the Warring States Periods (770 − 221 B.C.), there was a rise in swarms of various schools and thoughts, by virtue of whose work the experiences of their predecessors were summed up, perceptual knowledge about the nature, society and life was distilled and rationalized and raised to the level of theory. *Qigong* found its way to systematization and became an independent theoretical setup. For example, it was written in *Guanzi* that "The essence of life is the essence of *Qi*", "The heart is to the body as an emperor to his prone", and "*Qi* is what fills the body"."Preserving the innocent heart and cultivating the deposition" was put forward in *Mengzi (Mencius)*.The book *Xunzi* pointed out "keeping the mind blank to get tranquilized".The various schools came to hold their own theories on health preservation and brought about the concept of life essence, *Qi* (vital energy) and mental faculties —— the three treasures of the human body. "Exhale and inhale, to expel the stale and take in the fresh; a bear twists its neck, or a bird stretches its wings" written in *Zhuangzi* is also an examplary *Qigong* method for health preservation and treatment of diseases through limb movements in coorperation with breathing.

The *Qin*(221 – 207 B.C.) and Han (206 B.C. – A.D. 220) dynasties saw a rapid development of medical skills. The Yellow Emperor's Canon of Internal Medicine, the earliest medical classic extant in China, first took "*Daoyin*", "guidance of *Qi*" and "*Anqiao*" as important curative measures, pointing out a principle of health preservation " Be indifferent to fame or gain, be alone in repose, and take the various parts of the body as an organic whole". There is an account of the curative method by *Daoyin* in *Su Wen · Yi Pian Ci Fa Lun* (Plain Questions – On Acupuncture) which says "Patients with lingering kidney disease may face south from 3 to 5 a.m., concentrate the mind, hold back the breath, crane the neck and swallow *Qi* as if swallowing a hard object, for 7 times. After that, there would be a great amount of fluid welling up from under the tongue".

In 1973, a silk book *Que Gu Shi Qi Pian* (Fasting and Taking *Qi*) and a silk painting *Dao Yin Tu (Daoyin* Chart) of the Western Han dynasty (206 B.C. – A.D. 24) were unearthed from the Han Dynasty Tomb Mawangdui No.3 in Changsha, Hunan Province. The book records the *Daoyin* method for guiding *Qi* and the chart covers 44 coloured paintings presenting human figures imitating the movements of wolf, monkey, ape, bear, crane, hawk and vulture. This reveals that the Chinese began to teach *Qigong* through coloured atlas as early as the beginning of the Western Han dynasty.

The two outstanding medical scholars Zhang Zhongjing and Hua Tuo in the closing years of the Eastern Han dynasty (25 – 220) both referred to *Qigong*. In his great work *Jin Kui Yao Luo* (Synopsis of the Prescriptions of the Golden Chamber), *Zhang Zhongjing* stated that " As soon as heaviness and slugishness of the extremities is felt, start *Daoyin*, breathing exercises, acupuncture, moxibustion, massage with application of ointment to prevent obstruction of the nine orifices". The famous keeping—fit exercise *Wu Qin Xi* (Frolics of Five Animals) devised by Hua Tuo has passed down to the present days through generations.

During the Wei dynasty (220 — 265), the Jin dynasty (265 —420) and the Northern and Southern dynasties (420 — 589), *Qigong* had been developed not only in terms of health preservation but also treatment of diseases with out—going *Qi*. Zhang Zhan of the Jin dynasty listed in his work *Yang Sheng Yao Ji* (Essentials of Health Preservation) ten essentials, of which "thrifty of mentality", "preservation of *Qi*", "conservation of constitution" and *Daoyin* were all related to *Qigong*. Ge Hong of the Jin dynasty recorded, in his book *Baopuzi*, different methods of formulae for prolonging life span. Tao Hongjing of the Northern and Southern dynasties recorded in his book *Yang Sheng Yan Ming Lu* (Health Preservation and Longevity) a lot of ancient *Qigong* methods and theories. In "Treatment through Taking *Qi*" and "*Daoyin* Massage" of the book, he elucidated some methods of dynamic and static *Qigong*. In *Jin Shu* (History of the Jin Dynasty), an account was made on a doctor by the name of Xing Ling who became known to the whole country because he had cured, with out—going *Qi*, Lu Yi's mother of her illness" flaccidity— arthralgia—syndrome" from which she had suffered for more than ten years, and enabled her to walk. As a result, "There was a flow of people coming to see the wonder, either by land or by water".

Qigong was widely put into clinical application in the Sui

(581－618) and the Tang (618－907) dynasties. The books *Zhu Bing Yuan Hou Lun* (General Treatise on the Causes and Symptoms of Diseases), *Bei Ji Qian Jin Yao Fang* (Prescriptions Worth a Thousand Gold for Emergencies) and *Wai Tai Mi Yao* (the Medical Secrets of Official) have all included a wealth of *Qigong* therapies, mostly target-shoot (one method for one kind of illness) based on the overall analysis of symptoms and diagnosis.

In General Treatise on the Cause and Symptoms of Diseases, more than 260 therapies are recorded. While in Prescriptions Worth a Thousand Gold for Emergencies, the "Brahman Method of Indian Massage" and "Laozi Massage" are introduced in complete form among other *Qigong Daoyin* massage methods for health preservation. *Huan Zhen Xian Sheng Fu Nei Zhi Qi Jue* (Master Huan Zhen' Knacks in Taking *Qi*) of the Tang dynasty (618 － 907) describes the "Pithy Formulae of *Qi* Distribution", introducing the essentials and techniques of emission of out-going *Qi*. The anonymous book *Wunongzi* gives an account on how *Wunongzi* cured his bosom friend Yuzhongzi of his precordial pain by emission of out-going *Qi*.

During the period of the Song (960 － 1279), Jin (1115 － 1234) and Yuan (1271 － 1368) dynasties, there was an upsurge of exercises for cultivating "inner elixer" promoted by the Daoists. *Qigong* began to merge into these exercises. This promoted the development of therapeutic *Qigong*. For example, in the book *Sheng Ji Zong Lu* (The Complete Record of Holy Benevolence), which includes two parts —— *Daoyin* and *Fu Qi*(*Daoyin* and Taking *Qi*), are recorded abundant data of *Qigong*. Many *Qigong* descriptions could also be found in the works of the four eminent physicians in the Jin and Yuan dynasties. Li Dongyuan wrote in his book *Lan Shi Mi Cang* (Secret Record of the Chamber of Orchids), "Falling ill, the patient should sit still at ease to replenish *Qi*". Liu Wansu mentioned in his *Su Wen Xuan Ji Bing Yuan Shi* (Etiology Based on Plain Questions) the application of the "Six Character Formulae" in the treatment of diseases. Zhu Zhenheng stated in his book *Dan Xi Xin Fa* (Danxi's Experiential Therapy) that "Patients with syncope, flaccidity and cold or heat syndrome due to stagnation of *Qi* should be treated with *Daoyin* exercises". And Zhang Zihe put forward in his book *Ru Men Shi Qi*n (Prerequistite Knowledge for Physicians) that "*Daoyin* is one of the diaphoretic therapies", to mention but a few.

During the period of the Ming (1368 – 1644) and Qing (1644 – 1911) dynasties, the development of *Qigong* was characterized by deeper mastery and wider application of it by doctors. This enriched the medical books with *Qigong* literature and data. Abundant *Qigong* literature was included in *Yi Jing Su Hui Ji* (A Retrospective Collection of Medical Classics) by Wang Lu, *Wan Mi Zhai Yi Shu Shi Zhong* (Wanmizhai's Ten Categories of Medical Works) by Wan Quan, and *Gu Jin Yi Tong Da Quan* (The General Medicine of the Past and Present) compiled by Xu Chunpu. The great physician Li Shizhen had a deeper understanding of the ancient *Qigong*. He pointed out definitely in his book *Qi Jing Ba Mai Kao* (A Study on the Eight Extra-channels) that "The internal conditions and the channels can only be perceived by those who can see things by inward-vision". This famous thesis indicated the relationship between *Qigong* and the channels and collaterals.

Qigong has gained higher priority and more rapid development since the founding of the People's Republic of China. In 1955, a *Qigong* sanitorium was established in Tangshan. Inheriting the experiences of the predecessors and combining them with their own understandings in *Qigong* practice, Liu Guizhen and Hu Yaozhen wrote two books —— *Qi Gong Liao Fa Shi Jian* (The Practice of *Qigong* Therapy), and *Qi Gong Ji Bao Jian Qi Gong* (*Qigong* and Keep-fit *Qigong*), in which they introduced internal cultivation exercise, keep-fit exercise among many others, giving an impetus to the development of *Qigong* research in the whole country.

Since 1978, medical workers and *Qigong* masters all over China have made vigorous efforts to popularize *Qigong* among the broad masses for health preservation and disease prevention and gained satisfactory results. Some scientists and technicians have not only studied *Qigong* in terms of physiology and biochemistry from the point of view of modern medicine, but also conducted research on the physical effect of out-going *Qi* with multi-disciplinary efforts. A study on the nature and essence of *Qigong* has thus been initiated, and *Qigong*, as a new branch of science, has entered a new historic period of vigorous development. *Qigong* research societies, *Qigong* hospitals or departments have been set up in different provinces and municipalities for research, teaching and treatment. *Qigong* practice and study have become a common practice all over China. Morever, vast numbers of *Qigong* practitioners sum up and pool their experiences in time and in only a dozen of years, journals and magazines on *Qigong* such as *Qi Gong Za Zhi* (The Journal of *Qigong*), *Qi Gong Yu Ke Xue* (*Qigong* and Science), *Zhong*

Hua Qi Gong (China *Qigong*), *Zhong Guo Qi Gong* (Chinese *Qigong*) and *Dong Fang Qi Gong* (Orient *Qigong*) have emerged, and books such as *Qi Gong Liao Fa Ji Jin* (Outstanding Examples of *Qigong* Therapy), *Xin Qi Gong Liao Fa* (New *Qigong* Therapy), *Zhong Guo Qi Gong Xue* (The Science of Chinese *Qigong*) and *Qi Gong Yang Sheng Xue Gai Yao* (Principles of *Qigong* Regime) have been published.

1.3 Basic Principles of *Qigong* Exercise

1.3.1 Being Both Dynamic and Static

"Dynamic" and "static" are two general terms in *Qigong*, usually defined according to the body posture. The method that needs limb and body movements is referred to as dynamic *Qigong*, otherwise static *Qigong*. *Qigong* exercising calls for selection of methods which suit the health status of individuals. The practice of static *Qigong* is aimed at training and accumulating *Qi* to get functional *Qi* substantial in *Dantian*, and with further practice, to get *Qi* circulating through the *Ren* and *Du* Channels and all other channels (in a Taoist term, "opening the small circulation of *Qi*"). On the other hand, *Daoyin* is aimed at promoting the functional activities of *Qi* to guarantee free pass of it through all the channels of the human body, including the skeleton and extremities, to transfer genuine *Qi* directly to the diseased sites to get the disease cured.

No matter which of the two is practised, the principle "quiescence in motion and motion in quiescence" should be adhered to. When *Daoyin* is practised, while keeping physical movements going on, one needs to keep a serene mind which is concentrated on the effectiveness of limb movements and circulation of *Qi* along the channels and collaterals. When static *Qigong* is practised, the more serene and relaxed you are, the more you can feel the effectiveness of the circulating *Qi* along the channels and collaterals. A correct realization of the effectiveness of motion can help you concentrate yourself, expell distracting thoughts and raise the quality of exercising to a higher level.

1.3.2. Being Relaxed and Static Naturally

Relaxation, a principle in *Qigong* exercise, means both physical and mental, for only when one is relaxed mentally can he be so physically. However, relaxation here does not mean slackness or inattentiveness, but means relaxation with attentiveness, relaxation with tension and tension without rigidity, dominated by the conscious mind.

"Static" here means to keep a serene mind during *Qigong* exercise. Staticness is relative, there exists no absolute staticness. The so called "falling into static state" in *Qigong* is different from natural sleep and general rest. It implies a special static state with consciousness, or in other words, a special conscious state with staticness.

1.3.3 Coordinating the Will and *Qi* (Vital Energy)

The coordination of the will and *Qi*, as the term implies, means that in *Qigong* exercise, the will should follow *Qi* and vice versa. The practitioner should not put undue emphasis on exerting the will to guide *Qi*, which usually leads to forced "gentle, fine, even and long" breathing other than that acquired naturally through correct practice; nor should he force unnecessarily abdominal respiration which leads him to buldge his belly and throw out his chest on purpose, losing naturalness. Another deviation can be seen in the fact that when the motion of *Qi* is felt inside the body, the practitioner forces it by will to flow in a definite direction.This is also against the principle which needs the function to be formed naturally through practice.Xue Yanggui of the *Qing* dynasty (1644 − 1911) wrote in his book *Mei Hua Wen Da Pian* (Questions and Answers of Meihua) that "The tranquility of the mind regulates the breathing naturally and in turn , regulated breathing brings on concentration of the mind naturally; this is what is said the mind and breathing are interdependant and regular respiration producesa serene mind".

It is not advisable to put undue emphasis on realization of the flow of *Qi* either. The cold, hot, tingling, distending, itching, light, heavy, floating, deep or warm sensation experienced during *Qigong* exercising will go along a certain route. It is improper to pursue such kind of sensation intentionally or to exaggerate it, or force oneself to gain it.

In *Daoyin Qigong*, when selfmassage is carried out, it is stipulated that the will should follow hand manipulation and vice versa so as to realize the feeling of *Qi* under the hands, with breathing well coordinated. If the feeling is not quite tangible, one should not pursue it recklessly; it is enough just to concentrate the attention on the site under the hands.

1.3.4 Combining Active Exercise with Inner Health Cultivation

"Active exercise" means a series of procedures controlled by consciousness during *Qigong* exercising in terms of determination of a proper posture, adjustment of the body, internal and external relaxation, regulation of respiration, expelling of the distracting thoughts as well as hand manipulations. By "active exercise", is meant to practise *Qigong* under strong domination of consciousness by means of breathing and will. "Inner health cultivation" refers to the static state one falls into after active exercise, in which one feels relaxed and comfortable, with his will and breathing feeble and faint.

In *Qigong*, active exercise and inner health cultivation are done alternately and are interpromoting. For instance, one may have static inner cultivation after *Daoyin* has been practised or vice versa to achieve the effectiveness of "active exercise in static cultivation" or "static cultivation in active exercise", or in other words, "a combination of the two"; to raise the quality of *Qigong* exercising.

1.3.5 Proceeding in an Orderly Way and Step by Step

Qigong exercise needs to be proceeded in an orderly way and step by step. Be aware of the old saying "Haste makes waste". When *Qigong* or *Daoyin* is practised, priority should be given to the selection of practice methods. Through arduous training, the practitioner should enable himself to direct with consciousness the internal *Qi* to follow with the change of his posture, hand manipulation, respiration and will.

It is essential to learn some fundamental knowledge about it before practising *Qigong*. Remember that "Rome was not built in a day". People are liable to make such errors as, firstly, eager to achieve quick results, they want to cure their illnesses overnight and practise so much and with so much force as to cause fatigue, pain or soreness in some parts of the body or exacerbation of their illness, which make them daunted, thinking that the exercise is no good or some vicious thing has happened. The second is slackness, carelessness, and sloppiness in practice —— they let things drift, chop and change, go fishing for three days and dry the nets for two —— to them, success is surely too far away.

Therefore, to succeed in *Qigong* exercise, one needs to adhere to the requirements and practice earnestly. Efforts should be made to overcome all objective difficulties. If one is conversant with the knowledge of *Qigong* and practise it with perseverance, he is certain to obtain the anticipated results.

(Yu Wenping)

2 Three Kinds of Regulation in *Qigong*

2.1 Regulation of the Body (Adjustment of Posture)

Regulation of the body is also called posturization or adjustment of posture. It is especially important for the beginners of *Daoyin* or static *Qigong* to have a good command of proper posturization.

Four postures may be assumed in *Qigong* exercise —sitting, lying, standing and walking. Static *Qigong* usually requires a sitting, lying or standing posture while *Daoyin* can be practised in all the four. Postures for *Qigong* exercise presented hereof include sitting, lying and standing.

2.1.1 Sitting Posture

(1) Upright Sitting

Sit upright on a large even square stool. Ground the feet apart parallelly as wide as the shoulders. Bend the knees to form an angle of 90 degrees. Keep the trunk erect, the angle between the trunk and the thighs being 90 degrees. Rest the palms gently on the thighs. Bend the arms at the elbows naturally, look straight forward, tuck in the chin a little, let down the shoulders and draw the chest slightly inwards to keep the back straight, close the eyes and mouth naturally and apply the tongue aga the palate (Fig.1) .

(2) Sitting Cross-legged

Sit cross-legged on bed steadily with the two feet under the legs. Cushion the hips to raise them a little, with the body leaning slightly forward. Grasp the hands before the abdomen with the left above, the thumb of the right hand pressing *Ziwen* (the stripe joining the palm and the ring finger) of the left hand and the thumb and the middle finger of the left hand jointing together (Fig.2) .

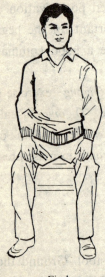

Fig.1

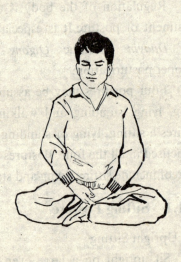

Fig.2

2.1.2 Lying Posture

(1) Lateral Recumbent Posture

Lie on bed in lateral recumbent posture (usually on the left side but it will do on either side) , the trunk being kept slightly bent. Rest the head on a pillow and lean it towards the chest a bit.

Keep the eyes and mouth slightly closed and the tongue against the palate. Put the hand of the lower side comfortably on the pillow with the palm upwards, and place the other palm on it to get the two palms closed. Or you can put the tips of the little, ring, middle and index fingers of the upper hand on the metacarpophalangeal creases of the corresponding four fingers of the lower hand, with the thumb of the upper hand resting on the outside part between the thumb and the index finger of the lower hand. Or you may place the arm of the above side naturally on the same side of the body. Stretch the leg of the lower side naturally, with the above bent and resting naturally on the lower one (Fig.3).

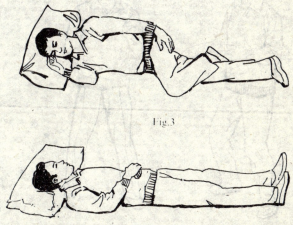

Fig.3

Fig.4

(2) Supine Posture

Lie on bed in a supine posture with the face upward and the neck straight. Stretch the extremities naturally with the two hands at the sides of the body or on the abdomen, overlapping one another. Keep the eyes and mouth slightly closed and the tongue against the palate (Fig.4).

2.1.3 Standing Posture

Stand on feet and set the feet apart as wide as the shoulders. Keep the head straight, the trunk erect, the chest slightly inward, the knees at ease and the arms raised and bent a little. Keep the fingers apart naturally, and hold the two hands close to the chest or the lower abdomen as if holding a ball (Fig.5) ;or

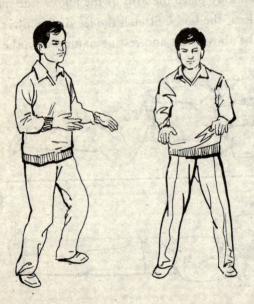

Fig.5   Fig.6

close the two palms in a way as if doing Buddhist greeting, or let the palms downwards (Fig.6) ; or let the hands overlap one another in front of the lower abdomen (Fig.7) ; or bend the right arm in front of the chest, palm upward to level with *Tanzhong* (Ren 17), while the left hand is held erect with the fingers pointing upward and the palm facing the thenar eminence minor of the right hand. This kind of hand position is called Heaven and Earth Palms (*Qiankun Zhang* gesture) (Fig.8).

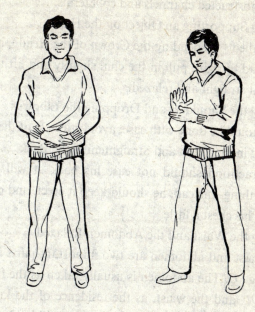

Fig.7 Fig.8

2.1.4 Essentials of Posturization

So far as the requirements for posture in *Qigong* are concerned, *Zun Sheng Ba Jian* (Eight Annotations on Health Preservation) cites a quotation from *Xin Shu* (The Book on Mentality), saying, "Sit on a thick-padded cushion, loosen the clothing, keep the back straight up, get the lips close to the teeth and prop the tongue against the palate, keep the eyes slightly open and stare at the apex of the nose". Although there is a variety of postures in *Qigong* exercise, the essential requirements for them remain the same.

(1) Loosening the Clothes

This step is essential to ensure a smooth flow of Qi through unobstructed channels and collaterals.

(2) Picturing Supporting an Object on the Head

Also called "Suspending the Crown of the Head", it needs to keep the head upright, pull in the chin slightly and lift the neck a little to get it straight and relaxed.

(3) Relaxing the Shoulders and Dropping the Elbows

This should be done with ease; avoid stiffness of the elbows.

(4) Drawing in the Chest and Straightening the Back

The practition should not ease his back at will or lean it against anything. Instead, he should keep it erect, and on this basis, draw in his chest a little.

(5) Keeping the Waist and the Abdomen Relaxed

The waist and abdomen are two important parts in training and guiding Qi. The abdomen is usually taken as the furnace for refining Qi and the waist, as the residence of the kidneys, the gate of life and the important pass of Qi and blood circulation. Relaxation of the waist and abdomen without slackness is helpful to the training and circulation of Qi.

(6) Contracting the Buttocks and Relaxing the Knees

Contracting the hips a little helps to straighten the spinal column; relaxing the knees permits free flow of Qi through the Three *Yang* and Three *Yin* Channels of Foot.

(7) Keeping the Toes Clutching the Ground

When the standing posture is taken, stretch the feet and let the five toes of each foot clutch the ground to keep the body as firm as Mount Tai (as stable as posssible).

(8) Curtain-falling and Inward Vision

It refers to dropping the eyelids to create inward vision on the spot where *Qi* is trained or circulates. *Yin Fu Jing* claims that the functional activities of *Qi* are determined by the eyes; *Ling Shu Jing* (Miraculous Pivot — the 2nd part of Canon of Medicine) holds that the eyes are the messengers of the mind, and the mind is the home of vitality. Eyes are of great importance in *Qigong* exercise. Curtain-falling and inward vision keep mentality undisturbed, turning off hallucination as well as sunlight. The eyes should neither be tightly closed nor left wide open; in the former, drowsiness may occur because of darkness and in the latter, vitality may be deranged because of too much light.

(9) Closing the Mouth and "Stopping the Ears"

Laozi (Laotzi) once said "Close the mouth to shut the gate". Closing the mouth here refers to closing the mouth slightly without clenching the teeth or tightening the lips, while stopping the ears means to focus one's hearing to oneself so as to be free from outside interference (inward-hearing).

(10) Sticking the Tongue against the Palate

Traditionally called "propping the palate with the tongue tip" or "tongue propping", it means to apply the tongue against the palate naturally and gently to communicate the *Ren* with *Du* Channels. In the course of practice, the strength of the tongue sticking against the palate will increase automatically and the tongue substance will be gradually pulled backward in accord. This is a phenomenom occurring in the course of *Qigong* practice and should not be pursued intentionally.

(11) When *Daoyin* is practised, the pushing, rubbing, kneading

and other hand manipulation methods as well as adjustment of the posture should be carried out along with the movement of the hands and with ease. Rigidity in movement should be avoided.

2.2 Regulation of Breathing

Regulation of breathing, also called inhaling and exhaling, breathing method, or venting and taking in *(tu na)*, is an important link in *Qigong* exercise. The ancients attached great importance to breathing exercises. A great many terms about breathing exercises can be found in books written in ancient times such as *Fuqi*(inhaling *Qi*), *Shiqi*(eating *Qi*), *Jinqi*(entering *Qi*), *Yanqi*(swallowing *Qi*), *Xingqi*(circulating *Qi*) and *Caiqi*(taking in *Qi*) ;as for breathing exercise, there are methods such as *Shangxi* (upper breathing), *Xiaxi* (lower breathing), *Manxi* (full breathing), *Chongxi* (blurted breathing), *Chixi* (lasted breathing), *Changxi* (long breathing) and *Shenxi* (deep breathing). The following breathing methods as required for *Qigong* practice are usually used.

2.2.1 Natural Respiration

Natural respiration is the ordinary breathing under normal physical conditions. Because of the difference in physiology between male and female and in the breathing habits of individuals, natural respiration can be further divided into natural thoracic respiration, natural abdominal respiration and the conbination of the two. Any of the above should be dominated by certain consciousness, performed naturally, and taken as the usual way of breathing in *Qigong* exercise.

2.2.2 Orthodromic Abdominal Respiration

It refers to trained natural orthodromic abdominal breathing exercises formed gradually under the guidance of the will through practice of natural respiration. To train orthodromic abdominal respiration, one employs a little consciousness to relax the abdominal muscles during inspiration to make the abdomen bulged naturally, and during expiration, uses some consciousness to get the abdominal muscles contracted. The contraction and relaxation of the abdominal muscles are intensified gradually and naturally through a certain period of practice. Forced exertion must be avoided. The orthodromic abdominal respiration tends to appear when one concentrates his mind on the navel.

2.2.3 Antidromic Abdominal Respiration

Antidromic abdominal respiration is the main breathing method used in *Qigong* exercises and in emission of out-going *Qi*. To get it, one uses the will to guide the abdominal muscles to contract and make the abdomen sunken during inspiration and , during expiration, relaxes the abdominal muscles gradually to get the abdomen bulged. Training in this way for a certain period of time will make antidromic abdominal respiration a natural one in *Qigong* exercises.

When antidromic abdominal respiration becomes more or less natural, it can be done in coorperation with contraction of the anus, which means to contract the anus and pudendum slightly during inspiration and relax them during expiration.

2.2.4 Other Breathing Methods

Apart from the above-mentioned main breathing methods, others that can be trained include long inhaling and short exhaling, long exhaling and short inhaling, nasal expiration and nasal inspiration, nasal inspiration and oral expiration and respiratory pause after expiration or inspiration. The selection of the breathing methods is based on the methods of *Qigong* exercise and the stage in practice. This will be described in detail when concrete *Qigong* methods are introduced.

2.2.5 Essentials of Respiration Training

(1) It is preferable to train mainly posturization first when one starts practising dynamic *Qigong*, *Daoyin* or static *Qigong*. Training of respiration should begin when one is skilled and natural in posturing. Otherwise adverse effects such as respiratory distress, emotional upset, chest stuffiness and headache may occur.

(2) The final goal of respiration training is to achieve deep, long, even and fine respiration. This is the result gained from long term practice; forced movements for lengthened or oppressed breathing should be guarded against.

(3) In *Daoyin* exercises, the movement of the hands is often done in cooperation with respiration. For example, pushing along the Three *Yin* Channels of Hands towards the fingertips is accompanied by expiration and pushing along the Three *Yang* Channels of Hand towards the shoulders and head is accompanied by inspiration. And this is defined by the run of the channels and collaterals, namely, the Three *Yin* Channels of Hand

run from the chest to the hands, the Three *Yang* Channels of Hand from the hands to the head; the Three *Yin* Channels of Foot from the feet to the chest and abdomen, and the Three *Yang* Channels of Foot from the head to the feet.

(4) Before starting respiration training, it is desirable to open the mouth to exhale, imagining that the obstructed parts of all the vessels are dredged and the turbid *Qi* is expelled from the body through expiration; then close the mouth to take in the fresh. Repeat the above inhaling and exhaling three times and then breathe naturally, adjusting it by will gradually to the respiration method desired.

2.3 Regulation of Mental Activities

Regulation of mental activities is also known as will control or thinking method. The training of the will is the most important link in *Qigong* exercise. *She Sheng San Yao* (The Three Gists of Regime) says, "Preservation of essence of life rests with cultivation of vital energy (*Qi*) which in turn rests with mental faculties. Mental faculty is to vital energy as mother is to child. So concentration of the mind would have vital energy consolidated while distraction of the mind would have it dispersed. He who only tries to save essence of life but neglects mental faculty knows the how but does not know the why". The heart governs mental activities. Here the relationship between essence of life, vital energy and mental faculty is stressed and great importance is attached to mental activities in *Qigong* practice.

1. During *Qigong* exercising, concentration of the mind on a certain part or a point of the body such as the Upper *Dantian*,

the Lower *Dantian* and the Middle *Dantian, Yongquan* (K. 1), *Laogong* (P. 8), the fingertips or palms, or on something or a spot fixed outside the body is known as localized mind concentration.

2. Another method is called directive mind concentration, which refers to the flow of *Qi* sensed when the mind goes with the movement of the hands or with *Qi* flowing along the channels, or sensed when the mind is concentrated on the two hands or on a certain part of the body.

3. Rhythmical mind concentration is the kind that occurs repeatedly or vibrates rhythmically or moves slowly with normal respiratory cycles, like the vibration produced by driving a pile.

4. During *Qigong* practice, one may think that he has as much strength as he could imagine. For example, he may imagine that he is strong enough to push a hill, to hold the sky or to pull nine oxen back by the tails. This kind of mind concentration is named power-strengthening mind concentration.

5. There is also suggestive mind concentration, referring to training of the thought, by which the movements are induced in coordination with the language, e.g., saying some words silently, meditating the results you wish to achieve by *Qigong* exercising.

6. The last kind is called representative mind concentration. While practising *Qigong* exercises, one may perform some imaginary movements and get *Qi* response in the long run. For instance, he may imagine he is stroking a ball, pressing *Qi*, instilling *Qi* and expelling unhealthy *Qi*, and he may feel *Qi* as hot as fire, as cold as ice, as sharp as a sword, or as soft as cotton.

7. Essentials of Training Mental Activities

(1) Mental activities should be coordinated naturally with respira-

tion and posture. For example, in dynamic *Qigong* exercises or *Daoyin*, mental activities must be adapted to the posture and the ascending, descending, opening and closing manipulations.

(2) Mental activities should be carried out naturally and progressively in a composed state of mind.

(3) Training of mental activity cannot go without "confidence". No matter what kind of mental activity you are exercising, you should be confident that you can realize the goal, though you should not expect unpractical quick results.

(4) Do not be overjoyed or frightened if something unexpected happens or you notice something by consciousness during exercising. Do not worry or talk about it.

2.4 Common Points

Qigong exercising often needs one to concentrate his mind on some points so as to train *Qi* or guide *Qi*, or to do massage on some points to activate and regulate the functional activities of *Qi* to cure diseases. Described hereof are the common body points used in *Qigong*.

1. *Baihui* (Du 20) It is the midpoint of the line extending over the vertex joining the apexes of the auricles. As it is also a converging point where the Three *Yin* Channels of Foot and the *Du* Channel joint, and located at the highest middle of the body, it is known as "the meeting site of all *yang*". Automassage of this point can cure headache, dizziness, vertigo, insomnia and prolapse of uterus or anus.

2. *Yintang* (Extra 1) Located at the midpoint between the eyebrows, it is the point of mentality and consciousness indicated for

headache, dizziness and diseases related to mentality and consciousness.

3. Upper *Dantian*   Also called "mud ball", it refers to the area between the eyebrows about 3 *cun* deeper than *Yintang* (Extra 1). As an important point in *Qigong*, the Upper *Dantian* is the site where vitality is stored and *Qi* is trained. Concentrating one's mind here during *Qigong* exercising helps to improve vitality and intelligence, but beginners generally should not try so.

4. *Taiyang* (Extra 2) It is located at the depression lateral to the external canthus and the tip of the eyebrow. Selfmassage of it can cure headache, cold, etc.

5. *Bizhun*   It is at the apex of the nose. Massage of this point can cure nasal obstruction and rhinorrhea.

6. *Fengfu* (Du 16) Located on the posterior midline of the neck, 1.0 *Cun* superior to the headline. Diseases caused by pathogenic wind or *Qi* can be treated by Selfmassage of it.

7. *Fengchi* (G.B. 20) Located at the depression outside the transverse muscle of the nape, lateral to *Fengfu* (Du 16). Selfmassage of it can cure cold, headache and conjunctival congestion, pain and swelling.

8. *Yuzhenguan*   On the superior border of the occipital protuberance, above *Fengfu* (Du 16). It is an important point for a smooth flow of *Qi* along the *Du* Channel in *Qigong*.

9. *Xuelang*   Located at the frontal border of the sternocleidomastoid muscle, lateral to the neck. Selfmassage of this point is effective for hypertention, vertigo and dizziness.

10. *Quepen* (St. 12) It is in the depression at the superior border of the centre of the clavicle, directly superior to the nipple. Selfmassage of this point can regulate the lung and stomach *Qi*,

and can cure cough, chest stuffiness, shortness of breath, etc.

11. *Tanzhong* (Ren 17) Located at the midpoint of the two nipples (the Middle *Dantian* is 3 *Cun* inside this point), it is a converging point of *Qi*.Selfmassage of it is effective for illnesses of the *Qi* system.

12. *Zhongwan* (Ren 12) At the midpoint between the navel and the xiphoid process. It is an important point for treatment of distension and pain of the abdomen, chest stuffiness, anorexia and other syndromes by means of *Daoyin* Selfmassage.

13. *Shenque* (Ren 8) In the centre of the abdomen at the umbilicus, it is the reservoir of acquired and congenital *Qi*, so both congenital and acquired diseases can be treated by *Daoyin* Selfmassage of this point.

14. *Guanyuan* (Ren 4) Also named *Dantian,* the point is located 3 *Cun* inferior to the umbilicus, on which the mind is often focused in *Qigong* practice because of its importance in training and reserving *Qi* and in treatment of congenital insufficiency of *Qi*.

15. Lower *Dantian* Located 1.3 *Cun* inferior to the umbilicus, about 3 *Cun* below the body surface, it is a common place for mind focusing in static *Qigong* and a place where motion of *Qi* is most obviously felt.

16. *Huiyin* (Ren 1) Located at the midpoint between the anus and pudendum, where the *Ren, Du* and *Chong* Channels originate. The beating that is often felt at this point during *Qigong* exercising is nothing but a sign of functioning of *Qi*.

17. *Jianjing* (G.B. 21) Located in the depression on the shoulder. Selfmassage of it to conduct *Qi* by will can regulate the activities of *Qi* in general and promote the circulation of

Qi in all channels. It is an important point for relieving pain in the neck, the arms and the lower limbs.

18. *Mingmen* (Du 4) It is located between the second and the third lumbar vertebrae, being an important point for treating decline of fire from *Mingmen*(the gate of life), impotence, nebulous urine, lumbar pains, etc.

19. *Changqiang* (Du 1) Also named *Weiluguan,* it is in the depression inferior to the tip of the coccyx. The conduction of *Qi* circulating through all channels by will starts right from here, a main point for conducting *Qi* in *Qigong* practice.

20. *Sanguan* It refers to the three important passes (points) for *Qi* circulation through the *Du* Channel, a collective term for *Weiluguan* or the coccyx pass (the site where *Changqiang* is located), *Jiajiguan* or the lumbar pass (lateral to the point *Mingmen)* and *Yuzhenguan* or the occipital pass (under the occipital protuberance where the point *Yuzhen* is located).

21. *Quchi* (L.I. 11) As the elbow is flexed at 90 degrees, the point is in the depression at the lateral end of the elbow crease. Selfmassage of this point is indicated for cold, headache, nasal obstruction, etc.

22. *Hegu* (L.I. 4) Located between the first and second metacarpal bones, it is indicated for headache, toothache, ear-ache, cold, etc.

23. *Inner Laogong (Neilaogong)* (P. 8) In the centre of the palm. As it is an important point for regulation of *Qi*, attention should be paid to the activities of *Qi* in this point when *Daoyin* is practised.

24. *Zusanli* (St. 36) Located 3 *Cun* below the outer depression of the knee. It is an important point for general improvement of

health and for treatment of abdominal pain and distension, cold and pain in the lower extremities, etc.

25. *Yongquan* (K. 1) In the depression of the sole formed when the toes are plantar–flexed. Being able to conduct the fire back to its origin, the point is important for training *Qi* and *Daoyin* massage.

2.5 Points for Attention in *Qigong* Exercise

1. It is essential for the beginners firstly to well understand the movements, the breathing method, the mental activities and the main points required for the exercises to be practised. Manipulation methods should be selected properly, and the points should be spotted correctly. Only when one is well acquainted with all these after initial studying for some time, can he go in for practising with unremitting efforts.

2. One must have his initiative fully displayed, be confident, determined and perseverant, and do the exercises in sequence and step by step. His work, study, life activities should be arranged properly to avoid distracting thoughts and anxiety during practice.

3. Generally speaking, the place for *Qigong* exercises should be one with fresh air and should be quiet. When doing the exercises indoors, quietude and good ventilation should be assured. Doing the exercises in draught or against fanning should be avoided.

4. Preparations should be made before the exercises. To avoid any possible disturbance to the functional activities of *Qi* and circulation of blood, one should first set his mind at rest, relieve himself, loosen the waist belt and take off the watch and spectacles.

Some *Daoyin* manipulations need to have the body surface exposed, and some concrete *Qigong* methods should be carried out faithfully in line with their essentials and points for attention.

5. Concerning the frequency of exercise, it is advisable to practise according to the requirements, as is required for the times of movement in some *Daoyin* exercises. The overall time for *Qigong* exercise is flexible, it should be set in accordance with the practitioner's constitution, the severity of his illness and the progress of the exercise. One should not force himrself to prolong the exercising time or increase the frequency. An optimum frequency or duration will always leave one with energy and interest, not tiredness.

6. Do not practise after eating too much or in hunger. Practising one hour after meal is desirable.

7. For the purpose of curing diseases, comprehensive measures may be taken, i.e., *Qigong* exercise may be performed in combination with medication or other therapies. As for women during menstruation, the time for exercise should not be too long; and too much mental activities towards the lower part of the body should be guarded against.

8. During exercise, some sensations such as hotness, distension, aching, tingling or numbness, itching, coolness, muscle twitch or a sensation of wormcrawl may occur. These are the normal manifestations of the functional activities of *Qi*. One should neither be nervous or frightened, nor try to get them out of curiosity. Just let things take their own course.

9. When *Qigong* is practised, sexual intercourse, smoking, drinking and intake of tea and hot or acid food should be moderate. Try to give up smoking gradually.

10. If one is suddenly panic-striken during exercise by a loud sound or accidental interruption by others, or peculiar phynomena occur during exercise, he should not be nervous and afraid. The proper way is to find out the cause of the panic and to set the mind at ease, and then continue the exercises.

11. *Qigong* exercise needs three steadiness —— steady start, steady performance and steady ending. Any careless start and ending may result in failure to conduct *Qi* back to its origin or lead to disorder of the functional activities of *Qi*.

12. Treatment of patients by emitting out-going *Qi* can only be carried out by those who have a solid foundation in training *Qi* and guiding *Qi*, and who have a good grasp of knowledge and experience in giving treatment by emitting out-going *Qi*, i.e., those who are qualified for such practice. The details for this are presented in chapter 4 of this book.

(Yu Wenping)

3   Various *Qigong* Exercises

3.1   Psychosomatic Relaxation Exercise (*Fangsong Gong*)

Psychosomatic relaxation is the basic exercise relatively easier to master compared with the other exercises in static *Qigong*. Relaxation, or to keep relaxed, quiet and natural, is the first thing to be done no matter static or dynamic *Qigong* is practised. Some psychosomatic relaxation can be taken as the rudiment to initiate *Qigong* exercises.

Methods

1. Posture

Any of the three postures —— standing, sitting or lying will do, however, no matter what posture is taken, the principle of being relaxed, quiet and natural should always be remebered. The muscles, the tissues of all the organs as well as the mind should be kept as relaxed as possible. The eyes can be either gently closed or slightly open.

2. Three—line Relaxation

The first line refers to the head, neck, shoulders and the lateral surface of the upper limbs; the second runs along the face, neck, chest, abdomen and the anterior surface of the lower limbs; and the third, the head, neck, back, waist and the posterior surface of the lower limbs.

When doing the exercises, concentrate the mind on the first part of the first line and say "relax" silently, and then on the next part. Do the same thing with all the parts on the first line in order. Then proceed to the second and the third lines. Repeat the procedure to the three lines in sequence 3 – 5 times with natural respiration for complete the relaxation exercises of the three lines.

3. Regional Relaxation

Concentrate the mind on one part of the body while saying "relax" silently in an orderly way from the head, the shoulders, the upper limbs, the back, the waist and the hips to the lower limbs. Repeat the procedure 3 – 5 times while breathing naturally.

4. General Relaxation

Take the body as a whole and relax it slowly from the head down to the feet, as if taking a warm shower. Do it with natural respiration.

5. Ending of the Relaxation Exercise

Stop saying "relax" silently after the static relaxation exercises. Resume the original posture and remain quiet for a while, and then rub the face and hands to end the exercises. Instead, one may also overlap the hands (the left under the right in male and vice versa in female) and rest them on the navel. Move the hands clockwise in ever-enlarged circles from the navel gradually to the flanks, for 36 turns, and counterclockwise from the flanks to the navel for another 36 turns. Then rub the face and hand to end the exercise.

Application

1. Psychosomatic relaxation as an exercise is generally used for health preservation or as rudiments for Qigong beginners. It is also used for treating many chronic diseases such as hypertension, neurosis, bronchitis, bronchial asthma, menopausal syndrome, gastritis, gastric and duodenal ulcers and chronic pelvic inflammation, and hypnotization.

2. Hypertension, headache, dizziness and other disorders are often treated with the "Three—line relaxation" method in combination with the Head—Face Exercise.

3. Diseases of the lung, stomach and heart are usually allayed with the "regional relaxation" method, with stress on relaxation of the diseased parts.

Points for Attention

1. The exercises can be done 1 — 4 times a day. The kind of psychosomatic relaxation to be taken is determined by the conditions of the individuals.

2. Psychosomatic relaxation is usually done with natural respiration and should be coordinated with mental activities (will). In general, the mind should be concentrated on a certain part of the body during inspiration and the word "relax" said silently during expiration.

3. Concentrating one's mind on a certain part of the body is an indistinct concept —— it seems that you are thinking of this part and it seems not. It is but natural for distraction to occur in the beginning.

4. Keep yourself light—hearted when doing the exercise. Stop the exercise temporarily whenever you are in anger or overexcited.

5. If you feel lethargic in a lying posture, you can try the sitting

and the standing.

3.2 Inner Health Cultivation Exercise (*Neiyang Gong*)

Inner Health Cultivation Exercise is one combining saying words silently with breathing. It acts very well on invigorating the functions of the digestive and respiratory systems.

Methods

1. Nasal Respiration

Take the lying or sitting posture, select either orthodromic or antidromic abdominal respiration. During nasal inspiration, put the tip of the tongue against the palate and direct *Qi* down to *Dantian* (1.3 *Cun* inferior to the navel) , thinking the word "I", then stop breathing, thinking the word "keep" or the words "I keep quiet" or "I keep quiet for the good of my health"; during expiration, the tongue is released. Start the exercise with saying less words, for instance, three, then five and then nine words the most.Inhale when you say the first part and exhale when you say the second part of the sentence.Hold the breath when you say the word in the middle.

2. Oral-nasal Respiration

Take abdominal respiration. Inhale by nose naturally and direct *Qi* down to *Dantian,* and exhale by mouth naturally to expel *Qi*, followed by holding the breath and saying words silently with the tongue stuck against the palate.Release the tongue when you complete saying the words and begin again for another round.

3. The same as that in ending off Psychosomatic Relaxation Exercise.

Application

1. The exercise is indicated for prevention and treatment of chronic gastritis, gastric ulcer, duodenal ulcer, chronic hepatitis, neurosism, hypertension, irregular menstruation, dysmenorrhea and other disorders.
2. Take orthodromic abdominal respiration at the initial stage of practice and change to antidromic when you are quite familiar with the exercise. Say silently no more than three words at the initial stage of holding–breath practice and increase the number of words gradually. Do not force yourself to hold breath or buldge your abdomen.
3. A warm sensation will be felt in the lower abdomen after long–term practice.

Points for Attention

1. Do the exercise 1 – 4 times a day, 10 – 60 minutes each time.
2. Take orthodromic abdominal respiration at the initial stage of exercise and change to antidromic when you are well versed in it. Be sure to say three words silently first when you start to hold the breath and increase the number of words gradually. Never force yourself to "stop respiration" or to bulge your abdomen intentionally.
3. Long–term practice will result in a warm or hot sensation in the lower abdomen.

3.3 Health Promotion Exercise (*Qiangzhuang Gong*)

Health Promotion Exercise is, by means of breathing and mind concentration on *Dantian,* to reinforce the intrinsic *Qi* to build up the health and prevent and cure diseases.

Methods

1. Natural Respiration

Sit cross—legged or take a standing posture. Take natural breathing and regulate it gradually to be quite ,even, fine and slow while concentrating the mind on *Dantian*. Mind concentration should be achieved in a vague manner, not strenuosly.

2. Deep Respiration

Take a cross—legged—sitting or a standing posture and, on the basis of natural respiration, slow down and prolong the respiration to make it quiet,fine, deep and even while concentrating the mind on *Dantian*.

3. Antidromic Respiration

Sit cross—legged or stand with antidromic respiration and concentration of the mind on *Dantian*. Pull in the abdomen and contract the anus during inspiration to instil *Qi* into *Dantian;* bulge the abdomen during expiration to descend *Qi* to *Dantian*.

Application

Health Promotion Exercise is helpful in building up the health and treating hypertension, neurosism, neurosis, coronary heart disease, arthritis, etc.

Points for Attention

1. Do the exercises 1 − 4 times a day, 10 − 60 minutes each time.
2. Fine, even, deep and long respiration can only be achieved through long−term practice and should not be pursued forcefully or by supressing breath.Stop exercising before you get tired.

3.4　Head−Face Exercise（*Toumian Gong*）

Head−Face exercise is aimed at beauty effect, health care and prevention and treatment of diseases by adjusting the channels and points at the head and face to promote the circulation of *Qi* and blood.

Methods

1. Preparation

Take the upright sitting or standing posture. Relax all over, apply the tongue against the palate,close the eyes slightly and get rid of distractions.

2. Pushing the Forehead

Put together the index,middle and ring fingers of the two hands and push the forehead with them from the midpoint of the eye−brows upward to the front hairline 24 − 50 times, then push from the midpoint of the forehead sidewards for 24 − 50 times (Fig.9) .Respiration should be fine and long. Push with more force while exhaling and less while inhaling. Try to feel the flowing of *Qi* beneath your hands while pushing.

3. Kneading−motioning *Taiyang* (Extra 2)

Put the middle fingers against the depressions lateral to the external canthi. Press and knead—motion counterclockwise for 24 – 50 times (Fig. 10). Refer to (2) for methods of mind concentration and respiration.

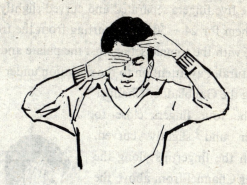

Fig.9

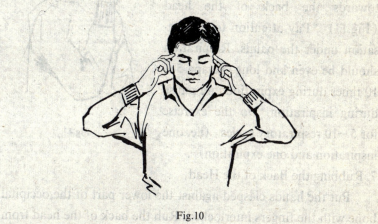

Fig.10

4. Bathing the Face

Rub the face with the two palms, starting from the midpoint of the forehead sidewards, then downwards, and then upwards along the sides of the nose back to the forehead. Rub clockwise with one palm and counterclockwise with another and vice versa for 24 — 50 times respectively with natural respiration. Try to get the feeling of *Qi* under the palms while rubbing.

5. Combing the Hair

Get the five fingers separated and curved slightly. Comb the hair with them for 24 — 50 times starting from the front hairline backwards, with the tongue set against the palate and the breathing kept natural. Pay attention to the sensation under the palms.

6. Sweeping the Gallbladder Channel

Get the four fingers close to each other and slightly curved. Scrape with the fingertips along the Gallbladder Channel from above the ears backwards via the frontal angle towards the back of the head (Fig.11). Pay attention to the sensation under the palms. Respiration should be even and long. Scrape 5 — 10 times during expiration and pause during inspiration. Do the exercise for 5 —10 respiratory cycles (i.e. one inspiration and one expiration).

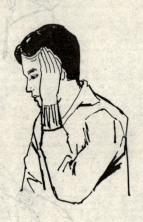

Fig.11

7. Rubbing the Back of the Head

Put the hands clasped against the lower part of the occipital bone with the fingers interlocked. Rub the back of the head from the top downwards for 5 — 10 times during expiration and stop rubbing during inspiration. Do this for 5 — 10 respiratory cycles, concentrating the mind on *Qi* activities under the hands (Fig.12).

Application

1. Head—Face Exercise is suitable for the young people to invigorate the skin and prevent wrinkles, and for the middle—aged and old to preserve health and prevent and treat loss of hair, hypertension, facial paralysis, headache, dizziness, cold, migraine, etc.

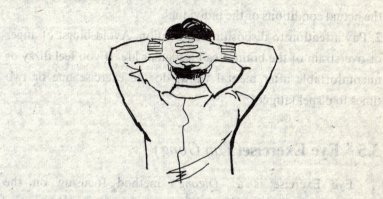

Fig.12

2. For good—looking purpose, put the stress on the three procedures ——bathing the face, pushing the forehead and combing the hair, with natural respiration and attention paid to the sensation induced by hand manipulation, and with agreeable imagination that your wrinkles have vanished, the Qi and blood are circulating perfectly, etc.

3. Those with headache and dizziness due to hypertension and neurosism should do more exercise of sweeping the Gallbladder Channel, massaging *Taiyang* (Extra 2) and scraping the back of the head. Pay attention to the sensation under the hands. Try to get the functional activities of Qi downwards during expiration

with hand manipulation. Stop the manipulation during inspiration. Avoid respiratory supression and violent rubbing or scraping.

Points for Attention

1. Do the exercise 1 − 4 times a day. Times of hand manipulations and the force used should be increased gradually depending on the actual conditions of the individual.
2. Pay attention to disposition cultivation. Avoid blurst of anger or overstrain of the brain. Lead a regular life. If you feel dizzy or uncomfortable after mental work, do the exercise one or two times to dispel fatigue.

3.5 Eye Exercise(*Yan Gong*)

Eye Exercise is a *Qigong* method focusing on the movements of the eyes, effective in regulating *Qi* and blood of the Liver Channel to soothe the liver and improve the acuity of vision.

Methods

1. Preparation
   Sit or stand erect, relax all over, look straight forward and expel distracting thoughts.
2. Moving the Eye Balls in "∞" Pattern
   Move the eye balls, imagining there is a flow of *Qi* inside the orbits. Start the eye movements from the point *Jingming* (U.B. 1) of the left eye. Move the eye balls along the upper side left orbit sidewards to the left canthus and then, along the lower

side of the left orbit to *Jingming* of the right eye, then along the upper side of the right orbit to the right canthus, then along the lower side of the right orbit to the left *Jingming* to form a "∞" pattern. Do the exercise this way for 8 times. Do another 8 times in the opposite direction starting from the right *Jingming*. Breathe naturally during the exercise. Direct the flow of *Qi* by will, and in turn the mind should follow the flow of *Qi*.

3. Pressing the Eyes to Guide *Qi*

Press with the thumbs on the internal upper corners of the orbits (the points Upper *Jingming*) and concentrate the mind here. Press backwards along the eye orbits while inhaling, and squeeze the eyeballs gently while exhaling, to get a soring and distending sensation in the eyes. Do this for 8 times (Fig. 13).

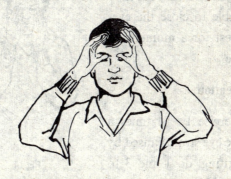

Fig.13

4. Bathing the Eyes

Close the eyes slightly. Make the flats of the four fingers rub each other and then rub with them the eyes from the inner corners sidewards for 24 times (Fig.14), with natural respiration and attention focused under the hands.

Application

1. The exercise is applied for keeping the eyes healthy and preventing and curing near sight, far sight as well as astigmatism in adolescence. Another function is to regulate blood and *Qi* circulation of the Liver Channel to soothe the liver and improve eyesight. Better results can be obtained when it is done in combination with the exercise of Soothing the Liver to Improve the Acuity of Vision.

2. It is also indicated for dizziness and blurred vision, dryness and discomfort of the eye, eye congestion, swelling and pain, as well as fatigue of the eye muscles in the middle-aged and old people.

3. It is desirable to close the eyes slightly and rest for a moment after the exercise.

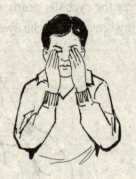

Fig.14

Points for Attention

1. Do the exercise 1 — 4 times a day. To relieve eye strain caused by reading or writing, do 1 and 3 to allay eye fatigue and protect eyesight.

2. Do not read in dim light. Order and wear proper spectacles timely when you are suffering from short or dim sight, or astigmatism. Pay attention to eye hygiene. Avoid eye fatigue.

3.6 Nose – Teeth Exercise(*Bichi Gong*)

It is the exercise for clearing the nasal passage and reinforcing the teeth and preventing tooth caries.

Methods

1. Preparation

Take a sitting or a standing posture. Get rid of nasal discharge. Be relaxed, quiet and natural. Breathe naturally.

2. Bathing the Nose

Rub the dorsal sides of the thumbs against each other till they are hot. Rub with them the sides of the nose gently up and down. Rub for 5 times during each inspiration and expiration for altogether 6 respiratory cycles (Fig. 15).

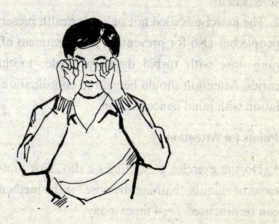

Fig.15

3. Kneading the Nose Apex

Put the tip of the middle finger of the right hand on the apex of the nose and knead it counterclockwise during inspiration and clockwise during expiration for 5 times each. Do this for 6 respiratory cycles.

4. Tapping and Clenching the Teeth

Get the upper and lower teeth tapping each other for 36 times and swallow the saliva. Always clench the teeth during defecation or urination, and loosen the teeth bite gradually when finished. Breathe naturally and concentrate the mind on the teeth so as to consolidate vital Qi.

Application

1. The Nose — Teeth Exercise can clear the nasal passage, protect the teeth and prevent dental caries. It is helpful to cultivate the habit of tapping the teeth and the habit of clenching the teeth during defecation and urination. Long—term practice will yield sure benefits.

2. The exercise is used not only for health preservation of healthy people but also for prevention and treatment of stuffy nose, running nose with turbid discharge, cold, toothache and dental caries. Attention should be paid to coordination of hand manipulation with mind concentration

Points for Attention

1. Do the exercise 1 — 2 times a day. For prevention and treatment of rhinitis, "bathing the nose" is the method of choice, which can be practised 2 — 4 times a day.

2. Hand manipulation should be gentle and deep—penetrating. Rough force should be guarded against to avoid skin injury.

3. Pay attention to oral hygiene. Expel nasal discharge before

practice.

3.7 Ear Exercise(*Er Gong*)

The exercise is mainly indicated for prevention and treatment of ear troubles. It also has the function of dredging the channels and improving the audition.

Methods

1. Preparation

Sit or stand with the whole body relaxed, inward—hearing turned on, mouth kept closed and the eyelids fallen. Breathe naturally and get rid of distracting thoughts.

2. Striking the Heavenly Drum (*Ming Tian Gu*)

Press the ears with the palms,the point Inner *Laogong* (P. 8) aiming opposed at the ear orifice and the fingers resting on the back of the head. Put the index fingers above the middle ones and then slip them down forcefully to tap the back of the head lightly for 24 times. You can hear rat—tat when doing this.

3. Pressing the Ears to Guide *Qi*

Press the ear orifices tightly with the palms and release them for ten times to compress *Qi* in the inner ears.Be sure to avoid forceful and violent pressing or releaseing. Though the pressing should be tight and releasing rapid, they must be done gently and moderately.

4. Massaging the Auricles

Pinch the top of the auricles gently with the thumbs and the index fingers and massage the auricles from the top downwards for 24 times , so much the better, to get them warm.

Application

1. Having the function of improving the audition, the exercise is indicated for health preservation and prevention of ear troubles.
2. For treatment of tinnitus, deafness and ear-ache, do the exercise in combination with kidney-replenishing exercises such as "taking black *Qi*", "rubbing the renal region" or "rubbing *Yongquan* (K. 1)", to render the effects more satisfactory.

Points for Attention

1. Do the exercise 1 − 2 times for health preservation, and 2 − 4 times for treatment of ear diseases. Do not exert too much force, especially when releasing the palms.
2. Pay attention to ear hygiene, keep constant inward-hearing for inner cultivation. If you have tinnitus, rub gently the ear regions with the two palms and move the head slightly before doing the exercise.

3.8 Neck Exercise(*Jingxiang Gong*)

It is a *Qigong* method of preventing and curing neck troubles, with the virtue of relaxing the muscles and tendons and activating the flow of blood and *Qi* in the channels and collaterals as well as lubricating the joints.

Methods

1. Preparation

Take a standing or sitting posture. Relax the neck, breathe naturally and look straight ahead.

2. Dredging *Fengchi* (G.B. 20)

Knead the point *Fengchi* gently with the thumbs 5 times during each inhaling and exhaling for altogether 14 respiratory cycles. Then with the thumbs and index and middle fingers clenched together, tap on *Fengchi* gently for 30 times.

3. Massaging *Tianzhu* (G.B. 10)

Bend the head forward slightly. Rub the back of the neck along its mid-line with the cushion of the four fingers of either hand from the top of the neck downwards for 7 times during expiration, and stop rubbing during inspiration. Do this for 8 respiratory cycles (Fig. 16).

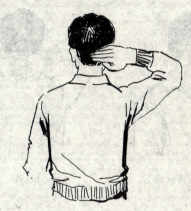

Fig.16

4. Massaging the Blood Waves (*Xue Lang*)

Close the four fingers of the right hand and rub with the cushion the blood wave regions on the side of the neck. During expiration, rub the left side (the left side first for the male and the right side first for the female), from under the jaw along the sternocleidomastoid muscle down to the clavicle; stop rubbing during inspiration. Do this for 14 respiratory cycles (Fig.

17).Then change hands and rub the other side of the neck.

5. Turning the Neck to Guide *Qi*

   Turn the neck counterclockwise for half a circle during inspiration and half a circle during inspiration for 8 times. Turn it clockwise in the same way for another 8 times.

6. Pulling the Neck

   Cross the fingers of the two hands to hold the back of the neck and pull the neck forwards during inspiration, at the same time thrust the head as backwards as possible and look upward. Relax during expiration. Do this for 9 respiratoty cycles (Fig. 18).

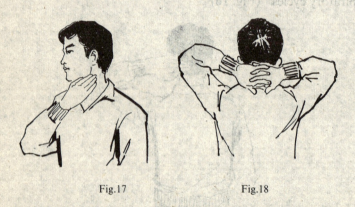

Fig.17   Fig.18

Application

1. The exercise is suitable for health preservation and effective for alleviating neck pain, cervical spondylopathy, stiff neck, fibrositis of the neck muscles, etc.
2. To treat hypertension, headache, dizziness or vertigo, methods 2 and 4 should be employed in combination with methods 5 and 6 described in 3.4, and with the exercise of Psychosomatic Relaxation.

3. For treatment of conditions such as servical spondylophathy and stiffneck, methods 3, 5 and 6 are recommended.

Points for Attention

1. Do the exercise 1 − 4 times a day, better to keep doing it once every morning.
2. The force exerted must be coordinative with the movements. The sphere of movements and the strength used should be increased gradually, the speed be controlled and coordinated with breathing.
3. Avoid resting the head on high pillows or bending the head over one's work too long. Those who have to take such a position in their work should choose several methods in this exercise for practice so as to relax the muscles and tendons, activate the blood and Qi flowing through the channels and collaterals, lubricate the joints, and relieve fatigue.

3.9 Shoulder − Arm Exercise(*Jianbi Gong*)

Shoulder − Arm Exercise, as a *Qigong* method to prevent and treat disorders of the shoulders and arms, can facilitate circulation of blood and Qi in the Three *Yang* Channels and the Three *Yin* Channels of Hand, subdue swelling, allay-pain, and lubricate joints.

Methods

1. Preparation

Take a standing or sitting posture, expel distractions, relax all over and breathe naturally.

2. Pounding the Shoulders and Arms

Make the left hand a hollow fist and pound the external, internal and anterior sides of the right arm from the shoulder to the wrist 3 − 5 times respectively. Then do the same for the left arm.

3. Dredging the Three *Yin* and Three *Yang* Channels of Hand.

Sit erect, place the right hand on the right thigh with palm supine. Massage with the left palm the internal side of the right arm from the uppermost, along the Three *Yin* Channels of Hand down to the palm (Fig. 19), simultaneously, exhale slowly with mind following the hand. Then turn the right

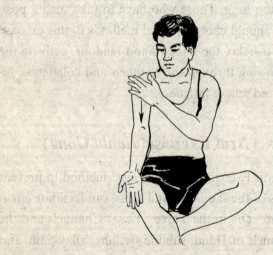

Fig.19

hand prone, and massage with the left palm from the back of the right palm along the Three *Yang* Channels of Hand up to the shoulder with inhaling and the mind following hand manipulation (Fig. 20). Do the above procedures for 7 times, followed by massaging *Hegu* (L.I.V. 4) with the left hand for 36 times.

Avoid holding breath during the exercise; relax the arms as much as possible. Dredge the Three *Yin* and Three *Yang* Channels of Hand of the left arm in the same way.

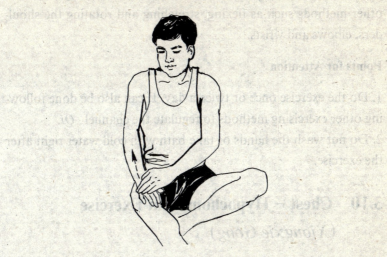

Fig.20

4. Kneading *Quchi* (L.I. 11)

Knead the point *Quchi* on the right arm with the left thumb for 36 times. Do the same to the left *Quchi* with the right thumb.

5. Kneading *Hegu* (L.I. 4)

Knead the right and left *Hegu* with the left and right thumb respectively for 36 times each.

Application

1. The exercise has the function of promoting the flow of *Qi* and blood in the three *Yin* and three *Yang* Channels of hands, relieving swelling and pain and lubricating the joints. It is applied to health preservation, indicated for conditions such as

aching—pain and numbness of the arm and shoulder, sprain and weakness of the limbs.
2. To treat arm and shoulder pain, do the exercise together with other methods such as flexing, stretching and rotating the shoulders, elbows and wrists.

Points for Attention

1. Do the exercise once or twice a day. It can also be done following other exercising methods to regulate the channel *Qi*.
2. Do not wash the hands or take bath with cold water right after the exercise.

3.10 Chest – Hypochondrium Exercise (*Xiongxie Gong*)

It is the *Qigong* method of preventing and treating disorders of the chest and hypochondrium, having the functions of relieving stuffiness of the chest and regulating *Qi*, Soothing the liver and lowering the adverse flow of *Qi* and relieving cough and reducing sputum.

Methods

1. Preparation
    Stand or sit, breathe evenly and relax all over.
2. Pushing—regulating *Tanzhong* (Ren 17)
    Conduct pushing massage with the index, middle, ring and small fingers from the suprasternal notch down to the xiphoid process for 36 times. Breathe naturally when doing this and concentrate the mind on *Qi* activities under the fingers.

3. Pushing the Chest to Regulate *Qi*

Do pushing massage with the right palm starting from the middle line of the chest leftwards for 5 — 10 times during expiration and stop pushing during inspiration. Do this for 10 respitatory cycles. Conduct the same with the left palm to the right side of the chest. Remember that mind should follow hand manipulation.

4. Rubbing the Hypochondrium to Descend *Qi*

This is done during expiration, with the two palms doing pushing massage starting from the armpit to the sides of the abdomen for 5 — 10 times.

Application

1. The exercise has the effect of relieving the chest stuffiness and regulating the flow of *Qi*, dispersing the liver depression and descending the up-adversed *Qi*, and reducing cough and sputum. It is applied to health preservation and prevention and treatment of stuffiness of the chest, chest pain, breathing disorders, profuse expectoration, dyspnea, etc.

2. In treatment of asthma and bronchitis, it is advisable to do the exercise in combination with Lung Regulating Exercise or the method of uttering *"Si"*.

Points for Attention

1. Do the exercise once or twice a day. It can also be done following other *Qigong* exercising methods, as a closing or auxiliary practice.

2. Be sure to keep fine, slow, even and natural breathing during the exercise. Never hold breath by force. Keep the muscles

relaxed.

3. It is desirable to find a place with fresh air to do the three steps of the exercise in order.

3.11 Abdominal Exercise (*Fubu Gong*)

The Exercise is defined as a common *Qigong* method of preventing and treating disorders of the digestive system. Ascribed to it are the virtues of strengthening the spleen and replenishing *Qi*, regulating the stomach and invigorating the middle—*jiao*.

Methods

1. Preparation

Lie supine, relax the whole body, apply tongue against palate and breathe naturaly.

2. Kneading the Abdomen to Reinforce *Qi*

Apply the right hand to *Zhongwan* (Ren 12) region and move the hand clockwise in circles to knead the abdomen for 36 times, then apply it to the navel region and move it clockwise and counterclockwise in circles for 36 times each.

3. Pushing the Abolomen to Promote Digestion

Do pushing the Abolomen with the four fingers or the whole palms of the two hands ,starting from the xiphoid process along the abdominal midline to the pubic symphysis for 36 times,and then do it starting from the xiphoid process, separating the hands and pushing them obliquely downward for 36 times. Carry out the manipulation during expiration; try to realize the sensation caused by hand manipulation.

4. Kneading *Dantian* to Strengthen *Qi*

Overlap the hands, the right above the left, and knead the midpoint of the lower abdomen with them for 36 times; then close the fingers in a pinch and tap the abdomen with the fingertips for 50 – 100 times.

Application

1. The exercise is suitable for health preservation of healthy people and prevention and treatment of abdominal pain and distension, disrrhoea, constipation, anorexia as well as colitis, gastritis, gastric and duodenal ulcers and other disorders of the digestive system.
2. Patients with diarrhoea and constipation can do the exercise following *Qi* Circlation Exercise to get better therapeutic effects.
3. For treatment of ulcers or colitis, it is desirable to precede the exercise with Inner Health Cultivation Exercise or Health Promotion Exercise.

Points for Attention

1. Do the exercise once or twice a day for preservation of health, and 2 – 4 times for curing illness.
2. Relieve bowels before practice. It is desirable to do the Exercise one hour after meal when you are neither full nor hungery.
3. Hand manipulation should be coordinated with respiration and mental activities, with proper speed and moderate strength. Never exert rough pressure or violent massage.

3.12 Waist Exercise(*Yaobu Gong*)

Waist Exercise, a method to keep the lumbar region fit, has the function of strengthening the muscles and bones and reinforcing the loins and replenishing the kidney.

Methods

1. Preparation

Stand erect, with feet apart as wide as shoulders; relax all over; and breathe naturally.

2. Moving the Waist to Strengthen the Muscles

Stand with arms akimbo and move the waist clockwise and counterclockwise 36 times each (Fig.21).

3. Pounding the Waist

Turn hands into hollow fists and pound with them the two renal regions and the lumbosacral portion 36 times each.

4. Rub the two palms against each other till they are hot, then rub with them the lumbar and renal regions from above to below until these regions get warmed.

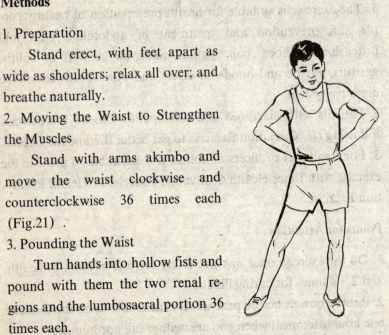

Fig.21

Application

1. The exercise is usually practised for health preservation and

prevention and treatment of lumbago, soreness in the waist, weakness of the knees, etc.

2. Those with lumbago due to kidney deficiency usually do the exercise in combination with such exercises as Nourishing the Kidney for Rejuvenation and Iron Crotch Exercise.

Points for Attention

1. Do the exercise once or twice a day.
2. Limit the frequency of sexual intercourse. The exercise can be done after practising other exercises so as to enhance the effect of waist training.

3.13 Exercise of the Lower Limbs (*Xiazhi Gong*)

It is an exercise to strengthen the waist and legs and to prevent and cure diseases of the lower limbs, with the functions of relaxing muscles and tendons and activating the flow of *Qi* and blood in the channels and collaterals.

Methods

1. Preparation
    Take a sitting posture.
2. Patting the Lower Limbs
    Bend one leg slightly and stretch another. Keep the hands stretched naturally and pat gently with the palm radiculus the stretched leg from the uppermost of the thigh down to the shank, 3 – 5 times. Then do the same on other leg.
3. Dredging the Three *Yin* and Three *Yang* Channels of Foot

Sit on bed, put the left hand near the base of the right thigh and the right hand on the external−posterior aspect of it. Conduct pushing massage along the Three *Yang* Channels of Foot downward to the foot while exhaling, mind following the hands (Fig.22). Then move the palms to the internal side of the foot and conduct pushing massage from the foot along the Three *Yin* Channels of Foot up to the uppermost of the thigh while inhaling, mind following the hands(Fig. 23). Do the pushing massage for 7 − 9 times.

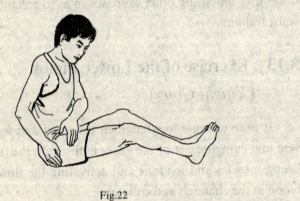

Fig.22

Application

The exercise has the functions of activating *Qi* and blood circulation in the Three *Yin* and Three *Yang* Channels of Foot, strengthening the waist and legs,and expelling wind and cold.
1. It is used for health preservation in healthy people and prevention and treatment of sciatica and arthritis.
2. For prevention and treatment of pain in the loins and knees caused by colddampness, weakness, numbness of the lower limbs and for relieving fatigue,the exercise can be done in combination

with *Hexiangzhuang Qigong* (The Crane Village *Qigong*) or Simultaneous Moving *Qigong*. (*Zifa Gong*)

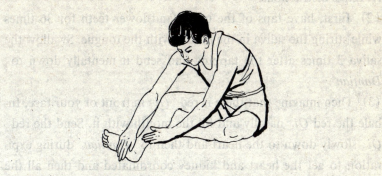

Fig.23

Points for Attention

1. To preserve health, do the exercise once or twice a day; to prevent and treat diseases, 2 – 4 times a day. Do it when you feel tired to relieve fatigue.
2. It is advisable to wear shorts during the exercise.

3.14 Heart Regulation Exercise
   (*Lixin Gong*)

It refers to the exercises regulating *Qi* and blood of the Heart Channel, effective for invigorating the heart and tranquilizing the mind, and promoting blood circulation and dredging the channels.

Methods

1. Taking "Red" *Qi*

(1) Preparation

Take a standing, a sitting or a lying posture. Breathe naturally. Expel distractions.

(2) First, have taps of the upper and lower teeth for 36 times while stiring the saliva in the mouth with the tongue. Swallow the saliva 3 times after the tapping and send it mentally down to *Dantian*.

(3) Then imagine that there is red *Qi* in front of your face. Inhale the red *Qi* nasally and fill the mouth with it. Send the red *Qi* slowly down to the heart and then to *Dantian* during expiration to get the heart and kidney coordinated and then all the channels of the body communicated with each other. Do this 7 −14 times. Resume to the preparatory posture to end the exercise.

2. Rubbing the Chest and *"ha"* *Qi*

(1) Preparation (Refer to 1−(1).)

(2) Tap the teeth and stir the saliva with the tongue as prescribed in 1−(2). As soon as the saliva is swallowed, put the right palm against the precardium and inhale slowly followed by slow exhale while pronuncing *" ha"* and concentrating the mind on *Qi* activities beneath the hand which rubs gently clockwise (Fig. 24) . Do this for 6 − 12 respiratory cycles.

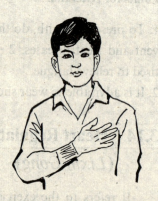
Fig.24

3. Invigorating the Heart and Guiding *Qi*

(1) Take the standing or the sitting posture, relax all over, breathe naturally, stick the tongue against the palate. Set the two palms against each other gently in front of the chest (Fig. 25) and keep still for a

moment while concentrating the mind on *Dantian*.

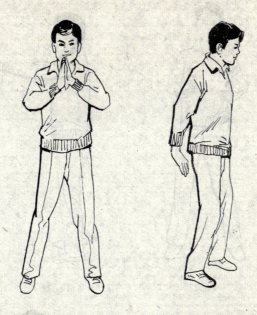

Fig.25 Fig.26

(2) Proceed from the last stance. Turn the palms outwards, the two arms stretching to the back along the sides of the body (Fig. 26). Keep still for a moment.

(3) From the last movement, turn the palms upwards and lift them beside the chest (Fig. 27).

(4) From the last movement, stretch the hands slowly forwards with force focused on the tips of the middle fingers. Abduct the palms with a little suppression on the thenar eminance major (Fig.28).

(5) From the last movement, clench the fists as if dragging some heavy things. Pull towards the back along the sides of the body (Fig.29).

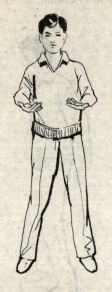

Fig.27

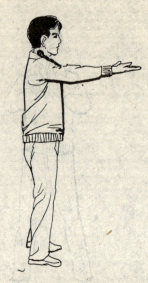

Fig.28

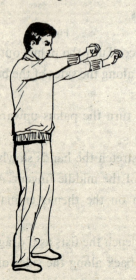

Fig.29

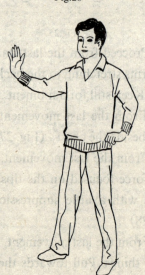

Fig.30

(6) Lift the right hand, as if holding a heavy thing, up to the chest. Set the palm upright and push it out right—forward (Fig.30). Pull the right hand back and lift the left hand as if holding a heavy thing and then push it out left—forward.

To end the exercise, return to the starting posture. Repeat the procedures 2 — 3 times.

Application

1. The exercise is applied in prevention and treatment of syndromes manifested by common or severe palpitation and precordial pain and insomnia as seen in coronary heart disease, hypertension, arrhythmia, rheumatic heart disease and cardiac neurosis.
2. Those who are feeble may take the sitting or lying posture.
3. Patients with deficiency syndromes had better practise "taking 'red' *Qi* " which has the effect of invigorating the heart, replenishing *Qi*, nourishing the blood and tranquilizing the mind. The exercise can also be carried out in combination with the method "invigorating the heart and guiding *Qi*" to activate the flow of *Qi* through the channels and collaterals. Patients with heart failure should put the stress on heart maintenance and do the exercise in combination with Inner Health Cultivation Exercise, concentrating the mind only on *Dantian*.
4. Patients with excess syndrome should take up "rubbing the chest and 'Ha' *Qi*", which emphasizes on purging pathogenic factors of the excess type and removing stasis. Then do the exercise in combination with "invigorating the heart and guiding *Qi*" to promote the flow of *Qi* along the Heart Channel.
5. For the purpose of health preservation, take "rubbing the chest

and 'Ha' Qi" as the chief method.

Points for Attention

1. Do the exercise facing south, 1 − 3 times daily.
2. Keep yourself light−hearted, lead a regular life and be on moderate diet.
3. Do the exercise in a quiet place to avoid fright. The duration and the frequency of exercise are decided according to the health status of the individual. The general principle is to have a sense of well−being after the exercise, free from fatigue.

3.15 Spleen Regulation Exercise (*Lipi Gong*)

It refers to regulation of the Qi and blood of the Spleen Channel, emphasizing on strengthening the spleen to replenish Qi and regulating the stomach to promote digestion.

Methods

1. Taking "Yellow" Qi
(1) Preparation
   Taking a standing or sitting posture, relax all over, breathe naturally, expel the distracting thoughts.
(2) Get the upper and lower teeth tapping each other for 36 times while stirring the saliva with the tongue. Swallow the saliva three times after the tapping and at each time send it down to *Zhongwan* (Ren 12) (the middle part of the gastric cavity) mentally.
(3) Imagine that there is yellow Qi in front of your face.

Breathe in the yellow *Qi*, fill the mouth with it and, during expiration, send it slowly down to *Zhongwan* (Ren 12) and then get it disperse through to the extremities and the skin and hair. Repeat the procedures 5 — 10 times before resuming the starting posture to end the exercise.

2. Rubbing *Zhongwan* (Ren 12) Area and "*Hu*" *Qi*

Take a standing or sitting posture. Put the right palm gently against the upper abdomen (*Zhongwan*) and exhale slowly. During expiration, rubbing the upper abdomen clockwise with the right palm (Fig. 31), and utter "*Hu*" at the same time. Do this for 10 — 20 respiratory cycles.

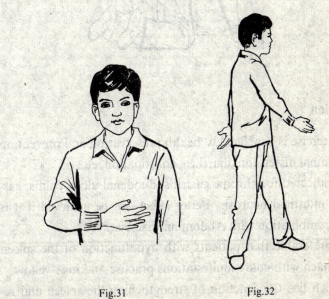

Fig.31   Fig.32

3. Dredging the Spleen and Stomach

(1) Take the standing posture, relax all over and breathe naturally. Get the arms swinging left and right with the waist as the

axle (Fig. 32), with the eyesight following the same direction of the swinging arms and the mind concentrated on the heels.

(2) Sit on heels, rest the palms on the bed and remain quiet for a while. Prostrate the upper part of the body with the hips raised and look back over the left shoulder like a tiger eyeing in the distance (Fig. 33). Then turn the head over the right shoulder and do the same. Repeat the procedures 5 times.

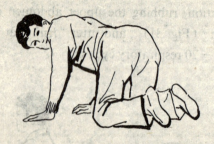

Fig.33

Application

1. The exercise is beneficial to health preservation and prevention of abdominal distension, diarrhea, constipation, etc.
2. It is indicated for chronic gastritis, duodenal ulcer, colitis, gastric and intestinal neurosis. Better effect can be achieved if it is done in combination with Abdominal Exercise.
3. It is preferable that patients with hypofunction of the spleen and stomach with cold manifestations practise "taking 'yellow' *Qi*", which has the function of strengthening the spleen and replenishing *Qi*. Those with heat syndromes of excess type should practise "rubbing *Zhongwan* (Ren 12) and '*Hu*' *Qi*", which has the function of promoting digestion, invigorating the stomach

and eliminating pathogenic factors. Patients with syndromes of either deficiency or excess type can take up "dredging the spleen and stomach" as well as Inner Health Cultivation Exercise.

Points for Attention

1. Do the exercise 1 − 4 times a day.
2. Lead a regular life. Don't eat or drink too much at one meal. Avoid doing the exercise when you are too full or too hungry.
3. The exercise is contraindicated in patients with bleeding and perforation in the stomach or duodenum.

3.16 Lung Regulation Exercise
(*Lifei Gong*)

The exercise is established to regulate Qi and blood of the Lung Channel, replenish the lung and regulate Qi, promote the dispersing function of the lung and send down the abnormally ascending Qi, and relieve cough and resolve phlegm.

Methods

1. Taking "White" Qi
(1) Preparation
   Take the standing, sitting or lying posture, relax all over, breathe naturally and dispel the distractions.
(2) Get the upper and lower teeth tapping each other for 36 times while stirring the saliva in the mouth with the tongue. Swallow the saliva 3 times after the tapping and send it mentally down to the chest, and further, to *Dantian*.
(3) Imagine that there is white Qi in front of the face. Inhale the

white *Qi* and fill the mouth with it. Send it slowly during expiration down to the lung and further to *Dantian*, and get it distributed to the skin and hairs of the whole body. Do this for 9 or 18 times, followed by resuming the preparatory posture to end it.

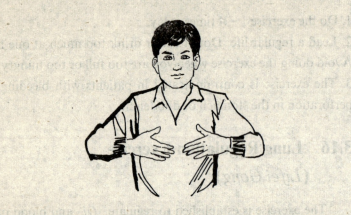

Fig.34

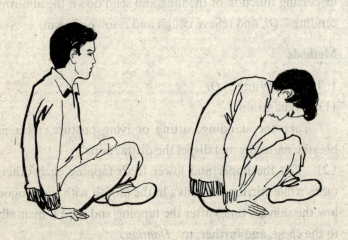

Fig.35   Fig.36

2. Rubbing the Chest and "Si" Qi

Take the standing or sitting posture. Put the flat palms on the respective side of the chest. Inhale slowly. Say "Si" during expiration with the two hands rubbing the chest in a rotative way (Fig.34). Repeat the procedures for 6 − 12 respiratory cycles.

3. Regulating the Lung and Guiding Qi

(1) Breathing with the Back Arched

Sit on cross-legs naturally, the palms pressing against the ground. Square the chest to get a deep inspiration. Hold the breath for a second (Fig.35), then arch the back and pull in the chest, and expire simultaneously (Fig.36). Do this 4 − 9 times.

(2) Regulating the Lung with Knee Movement

Stand with legs close together, put the palms on both knee-caps and rub the knee-joints slowly clockwise and counterclockwise 4 times each (Fig. 37). Inhale when rubbing the knees backwards and exhale when forwards.

Application

1. The exercise is suitable for keeping the lungs healthy and for prevention and treatment of chest stuffiness, chest pain, shortness of breath and profuse expectoration, and indicated for chronic bronchitis, pulmonary emphysema, bronchial asthma, etc.

2. The procedure "taking 'white' Qi", having the function of invigorating the lung and Qi, is effective for deficiency syndromes, while "rubbing the chest and 'Si' Qi", effective for excess syndromes. The exercise will give better effect if it is done in combination with Chest Exercise.

Points for Attention

1. Do the exercise 2 − 4 times a day, 10 − 40 minutes each time.
2. Smoking, drinking and raw, cold and irritating food are abstained from during the period of practice.
3. It is desirable for mild cases to practise in the park or woods where the air is fresh.
4. Those with infection of the lung should lie on the diseased side when a lateral lying posture is taken.
5. If you can not hold back coughing during practice, stop the movement to cough up the phlegm, then continue the exercise.

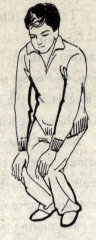

Fig.37

3.17 Liver Regulation Exercise
   (*Ligan Gong*)

This is an exercise with the function to regulate *Qi* and blood of the Liver Channel and to soothe the liver and subdue hyperactivity of the liver.

Methods

1. Taking "Green" *Qi*
(1) Preparation
    Take a standing, sitting or lying posture, relax all over, breathe naturally, expel the distractions and stick the tip of the

tongue on the palate.

(2) Get the upper and lower teeth tapping each other for 36 times while stirring the saliva with the tongue. Swallow the saliva three times after the tapping and each time send it down to the hypochondria and further to *Dantian*.

(3) Imagine green *Qi*. Inhale the green *Qi* by way of the nose and fill the mouth with it. Send it slowly down during expiration to the hypochondria and then to *Dantian*. Repeat the procedures for 8 or 16 times, then resume the preparatory posture to end the exercise.

2. Rubbing the Hypochondrium and "*Xu*" *Qi*

Take the standing or sitting posture. Put the palms against the ribs and inhale slowly. Say "*Xu*" during exhalation with the palms rubbing about the ribs (Fig. 38). Do the exercise for 10 — 20 respiratory cycles.

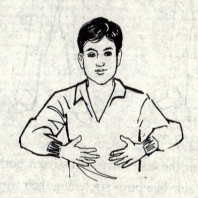

Fig.38

3. Soothing the Liver and Guiding *Qi*

(1) Stand relaxed and quiet, the two arms falling naturally on

sides, the palms facing downward, the five fingers raised slightly upwards and the palms pressing downwards with a little force, thinking that Qi has been directed to the centre of the palms and further to the fingertips. Press the palms downwards for 3 times (Fig. 39).

(2) Proceed from the last stance. Lift the two hands up to the chest with palms facing the front (Fig. 40). Concentrate the mind on the palms and push them outwards, then pull them back.

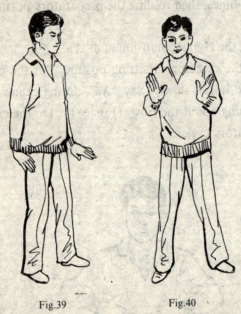

Fig.39   Fig.40

(3) Proceeding from the last movement, stretch both hands towards the respective side like birds stretching their wings, with the fingers tilted upward to throw the palms out parallelly to each side (Fig. 41). Guide Qi to the centre of the palms and further to the fingertips. Do the pushing 3 times.

(4) From the last movement, pull the palms back naturally to the chest, palms upward and fingertips pointing each other; concentrate the mind on the two palms and then turn them to face downward (Fig. 42). Push the palms downward to the pubic symphysis, directing *Qi* to the Lower *Dantian*. Turn the palms upwards to hold *Qi* and raise it up to the Middle *Dantian* (*Tanzhong*). Carry out the procedures 3 times, then drop the hands at the sides of the body to end the exercise.

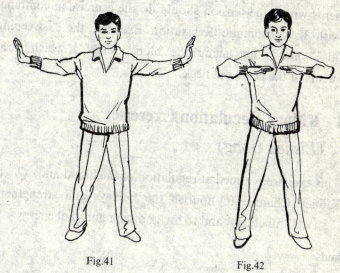

Fig.41   Fig.42

Application

1. Liver Regulation Exercise is applied in health preservation and prevention and treatment of dizziness, vertigo, bitterness in the mouth, dry throat, and fullness and stuffiness in the chest and hypochondra as can be seen in hypertension, neurosis, chronic hepatitis, cholecystitis, enlargement of the liver and spleen, etc.
2. For liver and gallbladder syndrome of the excess type, it is de-

sirable to take "rubbing the hypochondrium and '*Xu*' *Qi*", for the deficiency type, to practice "taking green *Qi*", and for treatment of both types, do the exercise in combination with "soothing the liver and guiding *Qi*".

Points for Attention

1. Do the exercise 1 – 4 times a day.
2. Avoid anger and keep a light heart during the exercise.
3. Patients with hypertension should do the exercise in combination with Psychosomatic Relaxation Exercise, the " sweeping methods" and " massaging the blood wave" , which need movements of the head and neck.

3.18 Kidney Regulation Exercise (*Lishen Gong*)

This exercise is aimed at regulation of the blood and *Qi* of the Kidney Channel to nourish the kidneys and strengthen *Yang* (vital function) and to invigorate premordial energy.

Methods

1. Taking "Black" *Qi*
(1) Preparation
   Take a standing, sitting or lying posture, relax all over, apply the tongue against the palate and expel distractions.
(2) Conduct teeth tapping for 36 times while stirring the saliva with the tongue. Swallow the saliva 3 times after the tapping and each time send it down to *Dantian* mentally.
(3) Imagine black *Qi*. Inhale it nasally and fill the mouth with

it. Send it slowly to the kidneys and then to *Dantian* during expiration. Do this for 6 — 12 times. Return to the preparatory posture to end it.

2. Rubbing the Abdomen and *"Chui"* Qi

   Stand or sit. Apply one hand against the lower abdomen and inhale slowly. Utter *"Chui"* during exhale, stroking the lower abdomen with the palm simultaneously (Fig.43). Do this for 10 or 20 respiratory cycles.

3. Strengthening the Kidney and Guiding Qi

(1) Stand erect, make fists and apply them against the soft parts at the sides of the waist and turn the waist counterclockwise and clockwise (Fig. 44) for 6 times each.

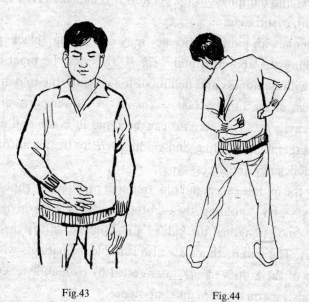

Fig.43   Fig.44

(2) Rubbing the Renal Regions

   Stand or sit, put the two hands on the sides of the waist and rub from above to below 36 times while concentrating the mind on the waist.

(3) Holding the Scrotum

Hold the scrotum with the right hand, apply the left palm to the pubes inferior to the pubic symphysis. Move the two hands up and down simultaneously 81 times. Change hands and do the same for another for 81 times.

Application

1. The Kidney Regulation Exercise is used for health preservation and prevention and treatment of pain along the spinal column, tinnitus, deafness, frequent urination, aversion to cold as well as coldness and dampness of the genitals. It is indicated for nephritis, neurosis, cystitis, etc.

2. Patients with kidney deficiency may do "taking 'black' Qi". "Stroking the abdomen and 'Chui' Qi" may be practised by those with dampness and itching of the genitals due to dampness and heat of the Lower–*Jiao* (*Xiajiao* — lower portion of the body cavity). The exercise can be done in combination with "strengthening the kidney and guiding Qi" to treat syndromes of both deficiency and excess types.

3. For the middle-aged and old, frequent practice of "rubbing the kidney" and "holding the scrotum" will help to invigorate Yang and strengthen the kidney and, constant effort yields sure success. The two methods are also suitable for patients with deficiency of the kidney–*Yang* manifested by pain and weakness of the waist, spermatorrhea and impotence.

Points for Attention

1. Do the exercise once in the morning and once in the evening, or up to 4 times a day.
2. Lead a regular life with temperance in sexual life. The young people should get rid of masturbation first so as to cure seminal or involuntary emmision.

3.19 Automatic Qi Circulation Exercise (*Zhoutian Zizhuan Gong*)

The exercise, otherwise named *Fa Lun Zi Zhuan* or *Xing Ting*, is, with the navel as the centre, to conduct circulation of Qi by mental activities and breathing in coordination with saying words silently.

Methods

1. Preparation

Sit or lie supine. Relax all over, breathe naturally, apply the tongue against the palate, and concentrate the mind on the navel.
2. Take the navel as the centre of a circle and move the abdominal muscles during inspiration, Qi following will. The moving starts during inspiration from the point right to and beneath the navel clockwise to the point left to and above the navel, while saying silently "The white tiger is hiding in the east"; then change into expiration and continue the moving to complete the circle while saying silently "The green dragon is hiding in the west". Move the abdominal muscles clockwise round the navel from the smallest circle to the largest for 36 rounds. Continue the moving in the opposite direction, i.e., starting from the point left to and beneath the navel upwards and rightwards to the point opposite the start-

ing point during inspiration, saying silently "The green dragon is hiding in the west". Complete the circle counterclockwise during expiration, saying "The white tiger is hiding in the east". Make the counterclockwise moving for 36 circles, from the largest to the smallest and eventually to the navel to end the exercise.

3. Beginners of this exercise may at first try to direct Qi to rotate by means of respiration and movement of the abdominal muscles. As soon as they are skilled they will be able to direct the intrinsic Qi to rotate round the navel only by will. This procedure is followed by rubbing the abdomen clockwise and counterclockwise for 36 times each to end the exercise.

Application

1. The exercise may be applied to rehabilitation, general health care of the aged and middle-aged and to disease prevention.
2. The exercise yields good therapeutic effects on diseases of the digestive system, such as gastric and duodenal ulcer, gastritis, enteritis and hepatitis. To treat syndromes of the excess type, such as abdominal distention or pain, impairment by overeating and constipation, move the muscles only clockwise for 81 times, and for deficiency syndromes manifested by diarrhea, poor appetite and weakness of the limbs, move only counterclockwise for 81 times.
3. Better effect will be achieved if the exercise is done together with the Abdominal *Daoyin* Exercise.

Points for Attention

1. Do the exercise 2 – 4 times daily for health preservation, and 4 – 6 times for treatment of diseases.

2. The exercise can be done flexibly besides regular practice hours. For instance, it can be done after work or study, or when the symptoms of a disease become severe, in which case it can be done until the symptoms improve. Persistent practice of this exercise may contribute a lot to regulation of *Yin* and *Yang* within the body.

3. Keep yourself relaxed and comfortable during practice. Forced holding of breath and mental strain should be avoided.

4. Be sure to defecate or urinate before doing the exercise. Any desire for defecation or urination may lead to diseases caused by mix—up of the clear *Qi* with the turbid.

5. Keep a proper diet. Overeating may cause stagnation of *Qi* while hunger may result in weakness of *Qi* in motion.

3.20 *Qi* Circulation Exercise (*Zhoutian Gong*)

Also known as Large Circulation of *Qi Da Zhou Tian*, Small Circulation of *Qi Xiao Zhou Tian*, and Exercise for Formation of Active Substance in the Body *Nei Dan Shu*, *Qi* Circulation Exercise takes an important place in health preservation and longevity. Only Small Circulation of *Qi* is described hereof.

Methods

1. Preparation

Sit cross—legged on a bed or upright on a stool with the chest pulled in, spinal column straightened, neck straight picturing supporting a light object on the head, shoulders relaxed, eyes slightly closed, and tongue stuck against the palate. Breathe evenly and concentrate the mind.

2. Take orthodromic abdominal respiration at first, and change to antidromic when you get familiar with the exercise. Respiration should be adjusted to be fine, gentle, soft and long. The mind is concentrated vaguely on *Dantian* (1.3 *Cun* inferior to the navel) . The fluctuation of the abdominal muscles should be coordinated closely with breathing, being lively and at ease.

3. After a certain period of training, you may feel a kind of warmness (*Qi*) in *Dantian*, which will be felt stronger and stronger. When such warm *Qi* has been accumulated to a certain extent, the flow of the hot *Qi* can be felt naturally;then you should have your will follow the flow of *Qi* from *Dantian* along the *Du* Channel via Huiyin (Ren 1) and the coccyx upwards directly to the vertex and to the cheeks, and then along the *Ren* Channel down to the chest, abdomen and eventually back to the Lower *Dantian*, to form the circulation so named Small Circulation.

4. Every time after the exercise, you should always concentrate the mind on Dantian for a while to get *Qi* back to its origion, followed by rubbing the hands and face to end the exercise.

Application

The exercise mainly applies to rehabilitation and health preservation.It is also taken as a rudimental exercise for treatment of chronic diseases.

Points for Attention

1. Do the exercise 2 − 4 times a day, 10 − 60 minutes each time. Increase the frequency and duration of sessions based on your

own conditions.

2. Before doing the exercise, loosen the waist belt, defecate completely and keep light hearted. Never do it when you are too full or quite hungery.

3. The effect can only be achieved naturally. Don't force yourself to gain quick results.

3.21 Exercise for Soothing the Liver and Improving Acuity of Vision (*Shugan Mingmu Gong*)

It refers to a set of exercises for dredging the liver–Qi to nourish the liver and improve the acuity of vision, with the functions of improving the eyesight, relaxing the neck and back muscles and relieving the muscular spasms of the eyes, and promoting recovery from fatigue. It has a satisfactory therapeutic effect on pseudomyopia of the shool children.

Methods

1. Preparation

Stand relaxed and quiet, place the feet apart as wide as the shoulders, drop the hands naturally at the sides of the body, picture supporting an object on the head, pull in the chest and straighten the back, relax the loins and knees, look straight forward, and breathe naturally.

2. Vision Regulation

Look straight forward first, and then look farther and farther until you can see no farther. Stare at a point for a moment and draw the vision gradually back to the nearest. Do this 4 times. Then look straight ahead as far as possible and simultaneously turn the eyeballs clockwise and counterclockwise for 4 times each. Breathe naturally during the procedures.

3. Turning the Neck and Moving the Eyeballs

   Look in the distance, turn the neck clockwise and counterclockwise for 4 times each, with the eyes following the movement of the neck. Inspire when the neck turns backwards and expire when it turns forwards (Fig. 45).

4. Throwing Out the Chest and Relaxing the Back

   Raise the arms to the chest with the elbows bent and palms towards the breasts. Draw the elbows backwards to throw out the chest and inspire at the same time; then relax the back and expire. Do this for 8 times (Fig. 46).

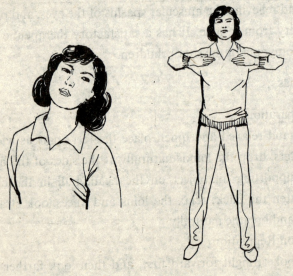

Fig.45   Fig.46

5. Pressing *Jingming* (U.B. 1) and Guiding *Qi*

Press with the thumbs the point *Jingming* (U.B. 1) near the inner canthus while concentrating the mind on the eyes. Press toward the orbits and then backwards during inspiration; squeeze the eyeballs gently during expiration while saying "*Xu*" (Fig. 47). The proper pressing should produce a sensation of soreness and distension but not pain.

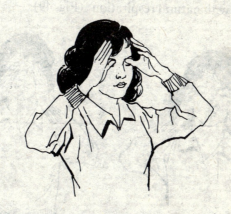

Fig.47

6. Pressing *Shangming* and Guiding *Qi*

Put the two thumbs on the point *Shangming* at the midpoint of the eyebow inferior to the upper orbit and concentrate the mind on the eyes. Press towards the orbit and its rear during inspiration; squeeze the eyeballs gently during expiration while saying "*Xu*". Try to get the sensation of soreness and distension without pain.

7. Pressing *Qiuhou* (Extra 4) and Guiding *Qi*

Put the two middle fingers on *Qiuhou* (Extra 4) which is a point one fourth from the outer side of the lower edge orbits, put the index finger lightly on the point *Sizhukong*   (S.T. 23) in the dent outside the tip of the eyebrow. Press the orbit backwards with the middle fingers during inspiration and, squeeze the eyeballs gently during expiration while saying "*Xu*" (Fig. 48).

8. Bathing the Eyes

Put the four fingers of the left hand on the left eye, right hand on the right eye, and rotate gently (the left hand clockwise and the right counterclockwise for 8 times and vice versa for another 8 times with natural respiration (Fig. 49).

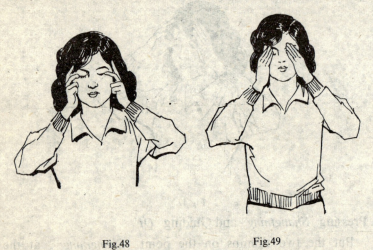

Fig.48　　Fig.49

9. Bathing the Face

Put the palms on the cheeks, rotate and knead gently in the same way and for the same times as that in bathing the eyes with natural respiration (Fig. 50).

10. Regulating *Qi*

Close the eyes lightly, bent the elbows and raise the hands in front of the abdomen, palms upward. Lift the palms slowly to the level of the eyes (Fig. 51).Concentrate on the eyes during inspiration, the two hands lifting to the point a fist from the eyes; then begin expiration while still concentrating on the palms, the two hands descending to the level of the abdomen. Do this for 8 times before dropping the hands at the sides as seen in the preparatory posture to end the exercise.

Application

1. The exercise mainly functions in prevention and treatment of myopia and astigmatism in adolescents, and in health care of eyes the in the young and middleaged.

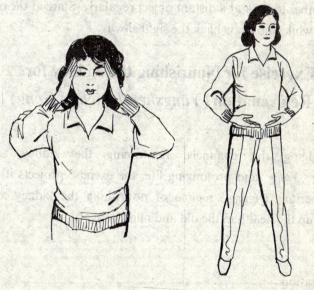

Fig.50　　　　　　Fig.51

2. There should be no distracting thoughts during the exercise. Mental activities and hand manipulations should be coordinated closely. There may be some kinds of sensations, e.g., depressing and tugging sensation between the palms and the eyes, itching in

the eyelids, and warmth and coldness in the eyes, which are normal effects of *Qi* activities. Keeping on doing the exercise and you are sure to be benefited.

Points for Attention

1. Do the exercise once in the morning and once in the evening.
2. Avoid overstrain of the eyes. If you have to read long, do some of the above exercises to protect your vision.
3. Do not get the distance between your eyes and the object too short, nor read in dim light or read lying or standing.
4. Remember to look at a distant object regularly. Stare at the object for a while and draw back the sight slowly.

3.22 Exercise for Nourishing the Kidney for Rejuvenation (*Yangshen Huichun Gong*)

Dredging the channels, reinforcing the kidney and tonifying *Yang* and prolonging life, the exercise projects itself as a superior *Qigong* regime of nourishing the kidney and building up the health in the old and middle-aged.

Methods

1. Preparation

Stand quiet and natural, with feet apart as wide as shoulders, hands hanging naturally, neck and spine straightened as if supporting an object on the head, knees relaxed and bent a little, toes clutching at the ground, tongue against the palate, eyes looking ahead but seeing nothing, breath even and mind concentrated on *Dantian*. Stand this way for 3 – 5 minutes (Fig. 52).

2. Contracting the Anus and Guiding *Qi*

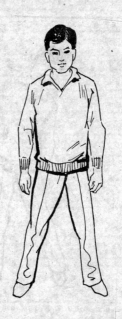

Proceed from the last stance. Take antidromic abdominal respiration. During inspiration, apply the tongue against the palate, shrink the neck and raise the shoulders, pull in the chest and abdomen, contract the anus, and at the same time lift the heels slowly to stand on tiptoe and direct *Qi* to circulate along the *Du* Channel up to the top of the head. During expiration, relax the anus, the abdomen and then the whole body, heels falling down slowly onto the ground while directing *Qi* along the *Ren* Channel down to

Fig.52

Dantian. Do the exercise 8 times. When directing *Qi* upwards, don't concentrate the mind too hard or repeat the directing, just think that *Qi* is circulating in a correct way no matter you feel it or not. Hypertensives may just think of *Dantian* and the point *Yongquan* (K. 1) without directing *Qi* to circulate upwards.

3. "∞" Pattern Shoulder Movement

Proceed from the last stance. Relax all over and breathe naturally. Turn the shoulders in a "∞" pattern with the waist as the axle. Male practitioners should turn the left shoulder first and female the right (Fig. 53). Turn the shoulders 8 times each or for the multiple of 8 based on the health status of the individuals.

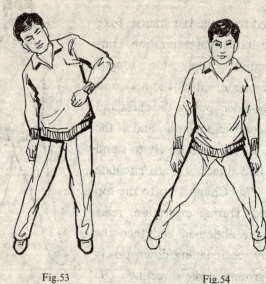

Fig.53 Fig.54

4. Rounding the Crotch and Shaking the Body All Over

Place the feet apart a little wider than the shoulders, contract the muscles of the legs slightly with the knees pulling somewhat toward each other to round the crotch (Fig. 54). Breathe naturally, close the eyes gently, relax the masseter, keep the lower abdomen in a state as if holding stools. Bend and straignten the knees alternately to lead the body to oscillate up and down with the upper and lower teeth clicking each other gently and the pudendum vibrating and closing and opening freely. Do this for 5 – 30 minutes each time or for a desirable duration according to one's health status.

Application

1. With its satisfactory effects for strengthening the kidney–*yang* and reinforcing the vital essence and *Qi*, the exercise is well suitable for the old and middle–aged people to preserve health. It is also used to treat climacteric syndrome in both male and female, impotence, prospermia, listlessness, lassitude of the limbs, greying of hair and premature senilism, hypomnesis and other syndromes.
2. The exercise can be done in combination with Waist–Abdomen *Daoyin* Exercise, Iron Crotch Exercise, etc.

Points for Attention

1. For health preservation, do the exercise once in the morning and once at night. Increase the frequency of practice if it is done to treat diseases.
2. Lead a regular life with temperance in sexual life.
3. Defecate before practice. Clothe yourself loosely, better in trousers of loose crotch.
4. Be natural and quiet. Avoid evil thoughts.

3.23 Exercise of Taking Essence from the Sun and the Moon(*Cai Rijing Yuehua Gong*)

1. Taking Essence from the Sun
(1) Preparation
   Stand quiet relaxed, and facing the sun with feet apart as wide as shoulders. Set the breath even, expel distractions.
(2) When the sun rises from the horizon, close the eyes, but not too tightly so as to see the soft and reddish sunlight. Inhale naturally the sun essence and fill the mouth with it mentally. Stop in-

haling and tranquilize the mind, and swallow the essence slowly during expiration down to *Dantian*. Do the inhaling and swallowing 9 times.

(3) Keep quiet and natural with the mind concentrated for a minute. Then move the body freely to end the exercise.

2. Taking Essence from the Moon

(1) Preparation

Select an open place with fresh air, stand quiet and relaxed, breathe naturally, expel distractions, face the moon.

(2) Close the eyes to see only the faint light of the moon. Inhale with both mouth and nose the moon essence slowly and fill the mouth with it mentally. Stop breathing somewhat and concentrate your attention. Swallow the essence slowly during expiration and send it down to *Dantian*. Do this for 6 times.

(3) Keep quiet for a minute, then move the body freely for a while to end the exercise.

Application

1. The exercise "Taking essence from the sun" can treat intolerance of cold due to *Yang* insufficiency, coldness of the extremities, weakness of the spleen and stomach, listlessness, etc. "Taking essence from the moon" applies to hyperactivity of fire due to *Yin* dificiency, lower fever, thirst and restlessness, feverish sensation in the palms and soles, pain in the loins and knees, etc.

2. For health care, you should set the session and duration of the exercise flexibly according to your own perceptibility to *Qi* activities.

Points for Attention

1. For health preservation, do the exercise "Taking essence from the sun" from three to seven a.m. on the first, second and third day of a month of the lunar calendar; do "Taking essence from the moon" from the fifteenth to seventeenth, 3 times each every month. Patients with insufficiency of *Yin* or *Yang* can do the exercises some other time besides the above-mentioned dates.
2. Do not do the exercise on cloudy, rainy or windy days.
3. If the symptoms have basically subsided, the patient should carry out the exercise in a way defined for health preservation.
4. Select a gracious environment with fresh air to do the exercise.
5. Be light-hearted. Avoid anger.

3.24 *Yang*-Recuperation Exercise (*Daoyang Gong*)

Yang-Recuperation Exercise is an exercise to induce *Qi* activities by means of posturing, breathing, mind concentrating and on-the-point finger-nail pressing, effective for invigorating the kidney, reinforcing the primordial *Qi*, and transformation of vital essence into *Qi*.

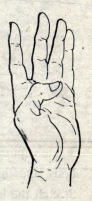

Fig.55

Methods

1. At night when the penis is erecting, lie on the right side of the body, bend the hip joints and the knees to touch the abdomen hard. Nip *Ziwen* (the stripe joining the palm and the ring finger)

of both hands with the thumbs (Fig. 55), the four fingers gripping the thumb tightly. Put the hands on the chest, close the eyes, rest the tongue against the palate, expel distracting thoughts, breathe naturally, and concentrate the mind on *Dantian*. Lie quietly this way for a minute.

2. Bow the waist slightly, with the middle finger of the left hand pressing the coccyx and the right hand still in a fist with the thumb nipping the stripe *Ziwen*. During inspiration, contract the anus, press the coccyx, bend the toes, make fist of the right hand, apply the tongue against the palate, and direct *Qi* mentally to circulate from the glans penis along the *Du* Channel up to the point *Baihui* (Du 20). During expiration, relax the whole body including the fingers, toes, anus and the tongue, and direct *Qi* to flow along the *Ren* Channel from *Baihui* (Du 20) down to Dantian. Facilitate *Qi* activities this way for 6 or 18 respiratory cycles (Fig. 56)

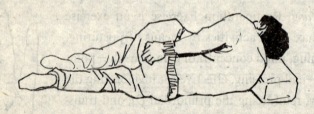

Fig.56

3. Lie supine with the arms laying naturally on each side of the body and the two hands in fists with thumbs nipping *Ziwen*. Stretch the legs. When inhaling, bend the toes of the feet hard, contract the anus, pull in the abdomen, apply tongue against the palate and make fists, then direct *Qi* hard by will to make it circulate from the glans penis along the *Du* Channel to the hind

head and further to reach the top of the head, and then, during expiration, direct *Qi* along the *Ren* Channel to *Yuanhai* (other name for *Dantian*) while easily relaxing the waist, legs, hands, feet, abdomen and anus. Repeat the procedures until the penis prostrates itself. Relax all over and concentrate on *Dantian* for a while before ending the exercise.

Application

1. The exercise is suitable to training *Qi* to preserve health. It is usually carried out when *Qi* is sufficient and *Yang* is exuberant, a time when one can transform essence into *Qi* and conduct the vital essence, *Qi* and spirit to the refiners (*Dantian*). Start the exercise as soon as the penis erects and stop when it is prostrated.

2. Doing the exercise can prevent nocturnal emission which is usually caused by hyperactivity of *Yang* due to insufficiency of *Yin*, breakdown of the normal physiological coordination between the heart and the kidney, failure in transformation of vital essence into *Qi*, and failure of the kidney in reserving essence. The practice of the exercise can restore normal coordination between the heart and the kidney and can transform vital essence into *Qi*. Do the exercise at night when the penis erects till it is prostrated. Or do it at night between 11 p.m. and 1 a.m. when sometimes the practitioner should try to get the penis erect and do the exercise. Practise in this way to prevent nocturnal emission.

3. Better effect can be obtained if the exercise is done in combination with the exercises such as "rubbing the abdomen", "holding the scrotum", "rubbing *Yongquan* (K. 1)" and Iron Crotch

Exercise.

4. If penis prostration is achieved after method 2, the practitioner can end the exercise without going on further.

Points for Attention

1. Never get evil thoughts during practice. Give up the bad habit of masturbation.
2. The youngsters may have two or three nocturnal emissions in a month, which can be taken as normal physiological phenomenon if there are no other discomforts. The condition can be improved after some practice of the exercise.
3. The practitioner should pay attention to hygiene and wash the pudendum constantly. Avoid wearing tight underpants. Lead a regular life with temperant sexual life.
4. The manipulations of pressing the coccyx, nipping *Ziwen* and making fists, contracting the anus, and resting the tongue against the palate should be closely coordinated with breathing and mental activities. The movements should be gentle and mental activities should be easy.

3.25   Vital Essence Recovering Exercise (*Huijing Huanye Gong*)

It is an exercise to send up the lucid *Yang* and send down the turbid *Yang* and to recover the sperm.

Methods

1. Preparation

When urinating, breathe evenly with one hand in a fist, thumb nipping *Ziwen*, the other hand holding the external genitals, the toes flexed towards the soles and the teeth clenched.

2. When some water has been passed, draw a sudden breath (with one hand in a fist, the thumb pressing *Ziwen* (Fig. 55) and the toes flexed) and simultaneously stop urinating and contract the glans and penis. Hold urine while direct *Qi* to *Mingmen* (Du 4, gate of life), then back to *Dantian*. Restart urinating and stop again in the same way. Do the procedures 2 or 3 times during one urination period.

Application

1. The exercise mainly applies to nocturnal emission and turbid discharge (sometimes looking like sperm) at the later stage of urination, discomfort of the urethra after urination, and distension and pain in the testicles and penis.
2. It is also indicated for relaxation of bladder sphincter and frequent urination.

Points for Attention

1. Do the exercise at urination.
2. Do not force oneself to hold urine or stools in daily life.
3. Give up masturbation. Do not be nervous on urination. Those suffering from nocturnal emission can do it together with *Yang*−Recuperation Exercise.

3.26 Filth—Elimination Exercise
   (*Dihui Gong*)

It is an exercise for elimination of the intestinal pathogenic factors.

Methods

1. Preparation

Take the sitting or lying posture. Relax all over, with the tongue against the palate, the eyes slightly closed, and the breath even.

2. Imagine that *Qi* whirls in by the upper orifice of the stomach and circulates in void to get genuine *Qi* to fill the intestines and drive the virulent heat—evil to wind from left to right and revolve through the intestine, and then come out of the anus. Then inhale and contrat the anus gently to close it. Conduct genuine *Qi* to wind from right to left in the opposite direction through the intestine and come out of the upper orifice of the stomach. Repeat the procedures 5 — 10 times.

3. After the exercise, concentrate the mind on *Dantian* for a moment to get genuine *Qi* back to its origin, then rub the abdomen, hands and face for a while to end the exercise.

Application

The exercise is indicated for heat syndrome due to retention of heat—damp evils and filthy *Qi* in the intestines, manifested by constipation, abdominal distension or pain, nausea and vomiting, and fullness and discomfort of the epigastrium.

Points for Attention

1. It is preferable to combine this exercise with that of "rubbing the abdomen". Rub the abdomen clockwise for 36 times before doing the exercise and counterclockwise for another 36 times after doing it.
2. Do the exercise 3 or 4 times a day. Increase the frequency if the symptoms are severe. As soon as the turbid *Qi* is driven out of the anus, reverse the exercise mentally to supplement genuine *Qi*.
3. The exercise is not suitable for deficiency syndromes such as constipation due to *Yin* deficiency, prolapse of rectum and tenesmic distention due to *Qi* deficiency.

3.27   Iron Crotch Exercise (*Tiedang Gong*)

Iron Crotch was regarded as an important exercise for training *Gongfu* of the lower part of the body in antient times. Modern times have seen great achievements of this exercise in terms of health preservation in the old and middle-aged and prevention and treatment of impotence, premature ejaculation, male infertility and other conditions. Its virtues to reinforce the kidney and invigorate yang, supplement *Qi* and nourish vital essence, and build up health are well established.

Methods

1. Pushing the Abdomen

Lie supine, relax all over, breathe evenly and expel distractions (similarly hereinafter), overlap the hands with the right above the left, and push the hands from the xiphoid process to the pubic symphysis (Fig. 57) for 36 times. Exhale slowly when pushing downwards with mind concentrated on the sensation induced by hand manipulation, This method is beneficial to strengthening the spleen and stomach and can direct genuine *Qi* to reach *Dantian*.

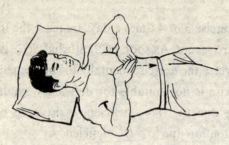

Fig.57

2. Pushing Separately on the Abdomen

Lie supine, and push with the hands from the xiphoid process separately to the sides of the abdomen (Fig. 58) for 36 times. Exhale slowly while pushing and concentrate the mind on the sensation preduced by hand manipulation. The method is beneficial to regulation of the stomach and promotion of digestion, and regulation of the flow of *Qi* to strengthen the spleen.

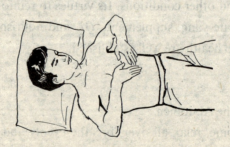

Fig.58

3. Kneading the Navel

Lie supine, overlap the hands (right above), and knead with pressure the navel clockwise and counterclockwise for 36 times each (Fig. 59), while breathing naturally and concentrating the mind on the sensation induced by the palms. The method has the function of strengthening the spleen and tonifying the kidney and warming *Yang* to dispel cold. Sometimes, a mass may be felt in the abdomen (usually below the navel), which is caused by stagnation of *Qi* and stasis of blood. This can be treated by persistent pressing and rubbing with the index, middle and ring fingers accompanied dy directing *Qi* towards it to make the channels and collaterals dredged and stagnation and stasis dispersed.

4. Twisting the Spermatic Cords

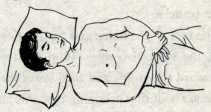

Fig.59

Take a sitting posture. Knead the spermatic cords lateral to the root of the penis with the thumb and the index and middle fingers and twist them left and right for 50 times, with the whole body relaxed and breath natural. Pay attention to the inductivity caused by hand manipulation, which is normally presented as aching distension without discomfort. Twisting this way functions in soothing the liver and activating *Qi* activities. Because the manipulation can irritate directly the spermatic cords, blood vessels, nerve tissues, and lymphatic vessels, their functions can be improved.

5. Kneading the Testicles

Sit and grasp both the testicles and the penis with the right hand, with the part of the hand between the thumb and the index finger forward and the testicles and penis exposed, holding the root of them tightly. Put the left palm on the left testicle and knead it for 50 times. Change hand and knead the right side for 50 times. Breathe naturally and concentrate the mind on the centre of the moving palm.

6. Rubbing the Testicles

Sit, with the surface of the index and middle fingers of both hands supporting the testicles of the respective side. Put the thumbs on the testicles and rub and twist left and right for 50 times.

7. Propping the Testicles

Sit, with the face of the index and middle fingers supporting the testicles of the respective sides. Prop the testicles with the fingertips up toward the groins and then lower them. Do this for 3 times. Inhale slowly during propping upwards and exhale slowly during lowering. Do not prop too hard, the proper manipulation should produce a feeling of bracing distension.

Kneading, rubbing and propping the testicles can facilitate the production of sperm and secretion of male hormone, being important hand manipulations of strengthening the kidney—*Yang* (fire from the gate of life) and replenishing the vital essence.

8. Swaying the Sand Bag

Stand erect, feet apart as wide as shoulders. Put the prepared sand bag and the gauze (with a slipknot) on the bed or on a stool. Grasp with one hand the penis and testicles, and get the slipknot looping at the root of the organs with an optimal degree of tightness, the two ends of the gauze equally long, pubes exposed. Then drop the sand bag slowly (Fig. 60), and swing it forward and backward for 50 times. Breathe naturally (Do not take abdominal respiration). The best effect is manifested by congestion and slight aching distension of the penis and testicles and slight aching distension and tugging sensation in the groins and even in the renal regions, with no pain.

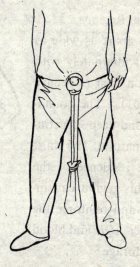

Fig. 60

This exercise gives irritation comprehensively to the male genital organs —— the testicles, epididymides, penis, scrota, spermatic cords and prostate glands, as well as the pudendal nerves, blood vessels and lymphatic ducts, to invigorate *Qi* and blood in the pudendum and improve the nutritional status and the functions of the genital organs. It is an exercise beneficial to nourishing the urogenital region, replenishing the vital essence and strengthening the kidney—*Yang*.

9. Pounding the Testicles

Stand erect, feet apart as wide as shoulders. Make hollow fists of both hands, pound with the back of the fists on both testicles alternately for 25 times each. The pounding should be gentle to achieve the best result —— a sensation of aching distension with no pain. The exercise can conduct the congested blood back to the kidneys to nourish the kidney—essence (genital essence).

10. Pounding the Renal Regions

Stand erect, feet apart as wide as the shoulders. Pound alternately with the back of the fists on their respective renal regions (Fig. 61). The pounding should be gentle and deep—penetrating, and the breath, natural. The waist is referred to as the residence of the kidneys; pounding this region can invigorate the kidneys and reinforce the waist, and can conduct *Qi* and blood back to the liver for storage.

11. Activating the Back

Stand erect, feet apart as wide as the shoulders. Make hollow fists, relax the joints of the shoulders, elbows and wrists. Sway the waist to lead one fist to pound the chest (palm facing the chest) and the other (the back of the fist) to pound

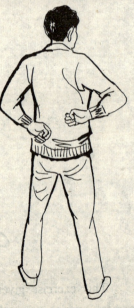

Fig.61

the region inferior to the scapula simultaneously for 50 times each (Fig. 62). This exercise can clear and regulate the channels and collaterals of the whole body to get *Qi* and blood circulating all over.

12. Turning the Knees

Stand with feet close together. Put the palms on the knees. Turn the knees clockwise and counterclockwise for 25 times each (Fig. 63). The exercise is effective in promoting the circulation of the channel *Qi* through the Three *Yin* Channels of Foot and the Three *Yang* Channels of Foot.

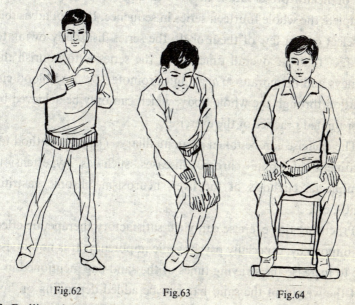

Fig.62 Fig.63 Fig.64

13. Rolling the Stick

Sit straight. Put on flat—sole shoes. Step on a round stick and roll it with both feet to and fro for 50 times (Fig. 64). The exercise has the effect of massaging *Yongquan* (K. 1), directing *Qi* downwards and conducting fire back to its origin (leading the ascending asthenic fire back down to the kidney).

14. Ending of Iron Crotch Exercise

Sit quietly with palms on the thighs for a while, then rub the face and hands and stand up and move the body freely to end the exercise. The ending procedures are essential for returning *Qi* and blood back to its origin to avoid dispersion and disorder of essence of life, *Qi* and the mental faculties.

Application

1. For health preservation in the old and middle-aged people, complete the whole fourteen series in sequence. It is not advisable to select only a few of them or do the series disorderly owing to the fact that the overall function of the series is to nourish the kidneys and invigorate *Yang* and promote *Qi* and blood circulation through the whole body, which can only be achieved by coordinated practice of the exercise.

2. The exercise can be taken as an auxiliary *Qigong* method for treatment of some chronic diseases such as hypertension, hemiplegia, cirrhosis of the liver, neurosism, chronic gastritis, colitis, etc.

3. Practising this exercise can yield satisfactory therapeutic effect on impotency, especially psychogenic impotency. It is not advisable to increase the swaying times of the sand bag mentioned in 8, but the weight of the sand bag can be added depending on how heavy one can bear. When the penis is able to erect after some practice, the exercise "grasping the penis" can be added, which means, when step 8 is completed, you may grasp the penis with one hand (glans penis exposed), and exert strength to direct

Qi and blood to the glans repeatedly for several times. The power of gripping and the grasping times can be increased gradually, but sliding of the hand up and down or swaying of the penis should be avoided.

4. If you are to treat prematural ejaculation or nocturnal emission, your penis may be easy to erect. When this happens, or when you feel an impulse to ejaculate, you should make efforts to dispel the distracting thoughts with firm will power and try to get the penis to collapse and the impulse to subside and then continue the exercise. There is one method to achieve this. First of all, make hollow fists of both hands and pound on the sides of the waist and the sacral region to get the erected penis collapsed; secondly, put together the index and middle fingers and support with them the penis at the frenum of the penis prepuce, with the thumb on the coronary margin of the glans penis, and knead and massage with force and at the same time, grasp the testicles and penis with another hand to pull them downwards for several seconds; release the two hands and repeat the kneading and pulling until the impulse subsides.

5. The non-ejaculatables may not practice swaying of the sand bag. Instead, rubbing the penis with the hands followed by holding the scrotum and testicles can be taken. Those suffering from infertility should double the practise of the procedures from 4 to 9.

Points for Attention

1. It is advisable to carry out the exercise under *Qigong* doctor's instructions. Never be too anxious for quick results. You may at first do the exercise for a hundred days without sexual in-

tercourse. The exercise is not suitable for those with post-operational scars and serious varicosis at the pudendum, vasoligation, acute testitis, epididymitis and otherwise.

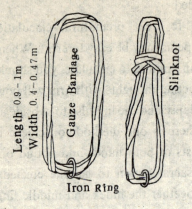

Fig.65

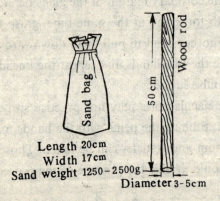

Fig.66

2. Get prepared with the sand bag, gauze, round stick, etc. The sand bag is made of cloth, 20 cm longth and 17 cm width, filled with 1250~2500g of sand and tied tightly at the opening. The gauze is 0.9~1m long and 0.4~0.47m wide, its two ends are

sewed up together and the whole gauze is made a ring (Fig. 65). The round stick is 50cm in length and 3 − 5 cm in diameter (Fig. 66) .

3. Go for defecation before practice. Do the exercise once or twice a day. You should feel no more than relaxed and comfortable during practice, although at first there may be a slight distending sensation in the groins and the testicles, which is the normal phenomenon and may disappear usually in six or seven days. If the reaction is severe, reduce the practice sessions.

4. To gain a better result, one should be light−hearted and confident,believing that the illness is surely to be cured. Don't put hasty for undue emphasis on penis erection, the proper way is to get rid of dread of impotence and to be active in practice and, when the kidney−*Qi* is vigorous, the illness is cured.

5. If you feel pain in the testicles, penis, pudendum, and the lower abdomen, there must be mild local damage and accumulation of *Qi* and blood which fails to disperse because you have done the exercise too much, or incorrectly,or you have carelessly increased the weight of the sand bag. These conditions can be corrected by reducing the practice sessions or holting the practice temporarily.

3.28 Daoyin Exercise for Ascending and Descending *Yin* and *Yang* (*Shengjiang Yin Yang Daoyin Gong*)

The exercise is designed to direct *Qi* to flow in a proper way along the Three *Yin* and Three *Yang* Channels of Foot and Three *Yin* and Three *Yang* Channels of Hand to keep *Yin* and *Yang* in equilibrium to cure diseases and prolong life.

Methods

1. Preparation

Stand erect, feet apart as wide as shoulders, hands falling naturally at the sides of the body, tongue against the palate, eyes looking straight ahead, neck straightened as if supporting an object on the head, shoulders relaxed and elbows dropped, breath even, and mind concentrated on *Dantian*.

2. Bent the waist slowly forward, hands in natural fists falling as low as possible in front of the feet. Simultaneously direct *Qi* of the Three *Yang* Channels of Foot from the head along the back, hips, lower limbs to the feet. Then straighten the waist slowly with fist clenched as if gripping something tightly; at the same time direct *Qi* of the Three *Yang* Channels of Foot to flow to *Yongquan* (K. 1), and continue to direct it along the Three *Yin* Channels of Foot up to the lower limbs, abdomen and finally the chest.

3. Proceed from the last stance. Turn fists into palms facing upward, lift the palms forward and upward until the arms are straight. Direct *Qi* of the Three *Yin* Channels of Foot mentally up to the chest, then along the Three *Yin* Channels of Hand to the upper limbs and finally to Inner *Laogong* (P. 8). Pull back the hands naturally, directing *Qi* of the Three *Yang* Channels of Hand to flow from Inner *Laogong* (P. 8) to Outer *Laogong* (P. 8), and along the Three *Yang* Channels of Hand upwards to the shoulders and head. Then clench the hands and direct *Qi* of the Three *Yang* Channels of Foot downwards. Make *Qi* flow this way for 36 circulations.

The movements should be integrated with breathing. Exhaling is required to cope with directing of *Qi* of the Three *Yang* Channels of Foot and the Three *Yin* Channels of Hand downwards, and inhaling to cope with directing of *Qi* of the Three *Yin* Channels of Foot and the Three *Yang* Channels of Hand upwards. Mental activties should follow the circulation of the channel *Qi*.

Application

1. This exercise can regulate *Qi* of all the Twelve Channels, applicable to health promotion as well as promotion of recovery of some chronic diseases under treatment.
2. Better results may be gained if *Daoyin* Exercise of the Twelve Channels is practised after practice of the above exercise.

Points for Attention

1. It is advisable to do the exercise after doing *Daoyin* Exercise for Dredging *Ren* and *Du* Channels in order to regulate *Qi* of the Fourteen Channels.
2. Do the exercise 1 − 4 times a day. It can be done before doing dynamic or static *Qigong* or all by itself, or in combination with *Daoyin* Exercise for Dredging *Ren* and *Du* Channels.
3. Conduct some free movement after doing the exercise.

3.29 *Daoyin* Exercise for Dredging *Ren* and *Du* Channels(*Tong Ren Du Daoyin Gong*)

Ren Mai (the *Ren* Channel or the Front Midline Channel) and *Du Mai* (the *Du* Channel or the Back Midline Channel) are the channels where all other channels converge. A free circulation of *Qi* in these two channels ensures that in all the others. The exercise described in this section is right for activation of *Qi* circulation in the two channels.

Methods

1. Preparation

Stand erect with feet close together, hands hanging naturally at the sides, chin tucked in as if supporting an object on the head, eyes looking straight ahead, breath got even, distractions expelled and mind concentrated on Dantian. Stand this way for a short while.

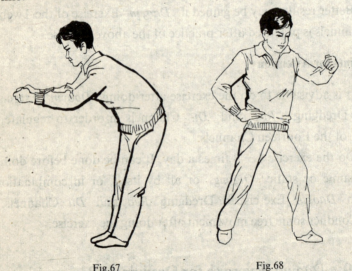

Fig.67   Fig.68

2. Activating the Coccyx (*Weiluguan*)

Bend forward at waist to form an angle of about 100 — 150 degrees. Get the hands gripped each other and stretched forward (Fig. 67). Look straight ahead but do not see anything, breathe naturally, induce *Qi* mentally from *Dantian* and accumulate it in the coccyx, and get the coccyx portion swing left and right for 36 times with the waist as the axle.

3. Opening *Jiajiguan*

From the last movement, make fist of the left hand and reach it out while the left foot stretches forward half a step; make the right arm akimbo, thumb backwards and the other fingers forwards to form a posture like a warrior pulling a bow. Then direct *Qi* mentally from the coccyx to the two points called *Jiajiguan*, and swing the body left and right for 36 times. Exchange hands and feet to swing for another 36 times (Fig. 68).

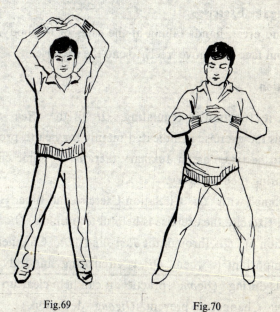

Fig.69   Fig.70

4. Dredging *Yuzhenguan*

Stand with feet apart as wide as shoulders. Raise the hands overhead and cross the fingers, palms upwards. Get the heels up and down as if pestling something for 81 times while directing

• 115 •

Qi mentally to float from the coccyx (*Weiluguan*) up to the back, *Jiajiguan, Yuzhenguan* and finally to the Mud Ball (the Upper *Dantian*) (Fig. 69).

5. Returning *Qi* to *Dantian*

From the last movement, make fists and raise them up to the level of *Tanzhong* (Ren 17) before the chest. Bend the knees to form a sitting posture, higher or lower relying on the constitution of the individual. Direct *Qi* from the Mud Ball (the Upper *Dantian*) along the *Ren* Channel down to the Lower *Dantian* (Fig.70). Concentrate the mind on the Lower *Dantian*.

6. Ending the Exercise

Stand erect, hands falling at the sides of the body. Rub the hands and face and move freely to end the exercise.

Application

1. With its function in regulating *Qi* of the *Ren* and *Du* Channels, the exercise is indicated mainly for health promotion. It may also be taken as an auxiliary therapy for some chronic diseases during their recovery.
2. Combined with *Qi* Circlation Exercise and Inner Health Cultivation Exercise, the exercise is helpful to training *Qi* and to the circulation of *Qi* through the *Ren* and *Du* Channels. What is more important is when *Qi* is circulating smoothly along the channels during *Qigong* practice, it can help clear up the *Ren* and *Du* Channels to prevent *Qigong* deviation.

Points for Attention

1. Defecate before practice.
2. The optimal time for practice is in the morning or at night after

dynamic or static *Qigong* is practised. If you cannot feel *Qi* activities, maintain only mental activities; the former can be achieved naturally by long-term practice.

3.30 Brocade Exercise in Six Forms
(*Liuduan Jin*)

This exercise, also called *Liuduan Gong* (*Qigong* in Six Forms), is designed to cultivate *Qi* and blood of all the channels and collaterals in general in a standing posture.

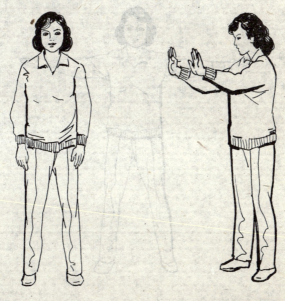

Fig.71 Fig.72

Form One   Stretching Out Hands to Shut the Cave Door
Set feet apart at shoulders width, the toes pointing inwards to

form inverted splayfeet, the waist and legs straight, eyes looking straight ahead, mind concentrated on *Dantian* and breath natural (Fig. 71). Lift the two hands with palms downwards to the two sides of the chest, and push forwards slowly as if shutting a door. Then strain the wrists and the ten fingers to exert traction to the tendons of the arms for 10 times (Fig. 72).

    Form Two   Stretching Arms and Shrugging Shoulders

    Proceed from the last stance. Abduct the arms and keep them at shoulder level, palms facing upward as if carrying a shoulder pole. Stretch arms backwards and simultaneously shrug the shoulders for 10 times (Fig. 73).

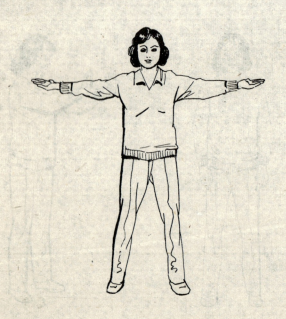

Fig.73

    Form Three   Pressing Gourd Gently

    Draw the hands back to the chest and drop them along the

chest to the sides of the legs naturally, palms facing downwards, fingers of them pointing at the opposite directions and bending upwards. Press downwards forcefully for 10 times (Fig. 74).

Form Four　　Bending Over to Touch *Dan* (Genuine *Qi*)

Keep the legs straight and bend the waist. With palms facing downwards, swing the arms crosswise and press the hands down and stroke for 10 times (Fig. 75).

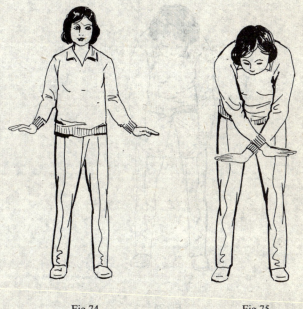

Fig.74　　　　　　　　　　Fig.75

Form Five　　Holding Mount *Taihang* by Hands

From the last stance, turn the palms upward as if to fish for something (Fig. 76) and lift them slowly to *Tanzhong* (Ren 17). Turn the palms upwards and stretch the arms slowly up

• *119* •

over the top of the head, arms apart at shoulders width. Then stretch the arms and palms forcefully upwards for 10 times (Fig. 77).

Form Six   Snatching the Belt with the Hand Alternately

Proceed from the last stance. Cup the hands slightly. Lower the left arm towards the front, and snatch as if to get something (Fig. 78). Withdraw the left hand to the chest and snatch with the right hand. Repeat this for 10 times.

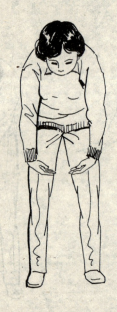

Fig.76

Application

1. This exercise is important for health recuperation and preservation. Better effect may be achieved if it is practised after static *Qigong* is done.

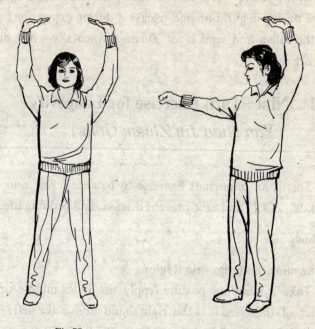

Fig.77　　　　　Fig.78

2. The exercise functions to promote the circulation of blood and Qi in the fourteen channels, regulating San−Jiao and strengthening the waist, legs and arms. It has satisfactory effect in treating pains in the loins and legs, soreness in the extremities and joints and dysfunction of San−Jiao.

Points for Attention

1. Do the exercise 2 − 4 times a day or after static Qigong is practised.
2. The practitioner should wear loose clothes when practising to avoid obstruction of Qi.
3. It is advisable to take nasal respiration with the tongue stuck

against the palate (It is allowable to press the tongue against the palate during inspiration and release it during expiration) . Swallow the saliva and send it to *Dantian* mentally when the exercises are over.

3.31 Nine—Turn Exercise for Longevity
   (*Yan Nian Jiu Zhuan Gong*)

This is an important Exercise to balance *Yin* and *Yang*, regulate *Zang* and *Fu*, prevent diseases and prolong life.

Methods

1. Kneading the Epigastric Region

Take a standing posture. Apply the index, middle and ring fingers of the hands (the right hand above the left) to the epigastric region and knead counterclockwise for 21 turns.

2. Pushing the Abdomen

Overlap the palms (the right above the left) and apply them to the epigastric region. Rotate and push them until they get to the pubic symphysis where they are separated and made to rub sidewise and upwards, back to the epigastric region. Repeat the procedure for 21 times.

3. Overlap the index, middle and ring fingers of the two hands, with those of the right above, and push along the abdomen downwards for 21 times.

4. Apply the right palm to the navel and rub it clockwise for 21 times. Do the same with the left palm counterclockwise for 21 times.

5. Stand with the left hand akimbo, thumb pointing the front. Push with the right palm from below the left breast towards the left groin for 21 times. Then, with the right hand akimbo, push with the left palm from below the right breast towards the right groin for 21 times.

6. Sit cross-legged after the pushing. Make fists with the two thumbs nipping *Ziwen* and put the fists on the knees. Throw out the left side of the chest and draw in the right to swing and turn for 21 times, followed by throwing out the right side and draw in the left and do the same movement for another 21 times.

Application

1. The exercise has the function of adjusting *Yin* and *Yang*, regulating the function of the internal organs, strengthening the spleen and stomach, and replenishing *Qi* and regulating the middle-*Jiao*. It yields good therapeutic results in treating gastric and duodenal ulcer, chronic gastritis, colitis, debility during convalescence, lassitude of limbs and poor appetite.

2. It is suitable for health preservation and rehabilitation of the old and middle-aged. The exercise can be done in combination with Regional *Daoyin* Exercise, Iron Crotch Exercise and others.

Points for Attention

1. Do it 2 — 4 times a day.

2. It is advisable to expose the chest and abdomen during practice. Respiration should be natural and attention should be paid to the sensation under the palms.

3. The manipulation should be gentle; violent rubbing or knead-

ing should be avoided.

3.32 Twelve-Form Sinew-Transforming Exercise (Yijin Jing)

Sinew-transforming exercise (*Yijin Jing*) is a salubrious method developed in ancient times. Tradition has it that the original intention of creation and introduction of it was to train the sinew. Literally, "*Yi*" means "transform", "*Jin*" means "sinew" and "*Jing*" means "method", by which the practitioner can turn his weak and flaccid tendons and muscles into strong and sturdy ones. Sinew-transforming exercise emphasizes coordinative training of movements, breathing and mental activities. During practice, the Qi and blood should be made to circulate appropriately at proper speed with no sluggishness or stagnation. The exersise is a set of highly salubrious one of its kind.

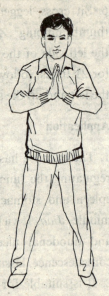

Fig.79

Methods

Form One   Wei Duo   **Presenting the Pestle**
1. Pithy Formula
   Keep erect when standing,
   Hold the hands before the chest as if praying,
   Set the breath even and keep the mind calm,

With the heart clear, soft and warm.

2. Posture and Essentials

(1) Step out with the left foot to set the feet apart at shoulder-width, hands hanging naturally, head and neck upright, eyes slightly open and looking straight ahead, tongue stuck against the palate, shoulders relaxed with elbows dropping, chest tucked in and back straightened, abdomen contracted and buttocks relaxed, knees at ease and slightly bent, and feet set steadily on the ground. Relax the whole body, breathe naturally, set the mind calm, restrain distractions.

(2) Turn hands into *Yin* palms (palms facing the ground) and lift them slowly to shoulder-level. Turn hands into *Yin-Yang* palms (palms facing each other) and draw them towards each other and close them before the chest. Bend the elbows slowly to get the fingertips pointing upward, the point *Shaoshang* (Lu. 11) on the two thumbs touching each other gentiy. Relax the shoulders and drop the elbows. Take abdominal respiration and keep *Qi* down to *Dantian*. You may feel the flow of *Qi* at this time. Have your mind follow the flow of *Qi* and, during inhaling, guide *Qi* to flow out of the fingertips, enter the nostrils and go down to *Dantian*. During exhaling, guide *Qi* from *Dantian* to the chest and then to the palms along the Three *Yin* Channels of Hand to fill the fingertips (Fig.79).

Form Two   Carrying A Monster-Vanquishing Pole Across on the Shoulders

1. Pithy Formula

　　Stand on tiptoe upright,
　　Stretch the two arms wide,
　　Set the mind quiet,

the breath even,
And the eyes and mouth widely open
as if stunned.

2. Posture and Essentials

(1) Proceed from the last stance.

(2) Turn both palms slowly into *Yin* palms (palms facing the ground) and move them sidewise respectively to form a straight parallel line. Simultaneously, lift the heels slightly to stand on tiptoe (when skilled one may touch the ground with only the big toes). Concentrate the mind and look fixedly ahead, with the chest tucked in and the back straightened, abdomen contracted and buttocks relaxed, and tongue stuck against the palate (Fig. 80). Breathe naturally, concentrating the mind on *Laogong* (P. 8) and on the toes. Turn natural respiration into abdominal

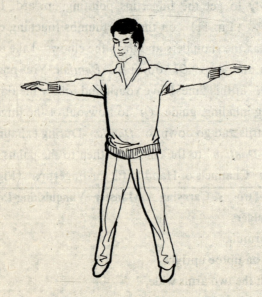

Fig.80

when you get familiar with the exercise, and concentrate the mind on *Laogong* (P. 8) when inhaling, and on the big toes of the feet when exhaling.

Form Three   Holding the Heavenly Gate with the Palms

1. Pithy Formula

　　Hold the heavenly gate with the palms and look inwardly up,
　　Stand on front sole and upright.
　　The whole body is planted as a sturdy pine,
　　And the teeth are clentched tight.
　　Saliva gushes as the tongue is pressed against the palate,
　　With nasal breathing the mind is set quiet.
　　As the two fists are slowly lowered,
　　Strength is exerted as if pulling a heavy weight.

2. Posture and Essentials

(1) Proceed from the last stance.

(2) Move both hands (in *Yin* palms) slowly up from their respective side to draw an arch. Turn the *Yin* palms into *Yang* (palms facing upwards), with fingers of the two hands pointing each other just above *Tianmen* (2 *Cun* up above the front hair line), as if holding the heavenly gate. Lift the heels simultaneously to stand on tiptoe, the heels inclining slightly sidewise to set the "*Yinqiao* Storehouse" (the point *Huiyin*, Ren 1) closed, at the same time set the point *Huiyang* (U.B. 35) open. Clench the teeth, rest the tongue against the palate. Apply inward-vision to stare through *Tianmen* (Heavenly Gate) at the space between the two hands (Fig. 81).

(3) Make fists, the arms falling slowly along the original arc until they are in the stance "Carrying a Monster-vanquishing Pole Across on the Shoulders", then you should turn nasal

inhalingmouth exhaling into nasal respiration and guide *Qi* down to *Dantian*. The respiration should be fine, even, long, slow and continuous. During inhaling, the mind is set on *Dantian* and gradually shifted to between the two palms during inhaling. When *Qi* is in circulation, let the mind follow *Qi*.

Form Four   Plucking and Reseting Stars

1. Pithy Formula

   Over the head hold the sky with one palm,
   Stare at Inner *Laogong* in calm.
   Inhale by nose and exhale by mouth,
   Attentively shift the eyesight to another palm.

2. Posture and Essentials

(1) Proceed from the last stance.

(2) Lift the right hand slowly to about one fist over the forehead. Lower the left hand simultaneously and rest the back of it on the left side of the small of the back. Concentrate the sight on Inner *Laogong* (P. 8) of the right palm (Fig. 82).

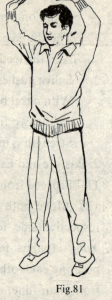

Fig.81

(3) Lift the left hand to about one fist off the forehead and lower the right one and rest its back on the right side of the small of the back. Concentrate the sight on *Laogong* (P. 8) of the left palm. Take nasal inhaling and mouth exhaling and adjust the breath even. While concentrating the mind on *Laogong* (P. 8) of the raised hand, make Inner *Laogong* (P. 8) of the raised hand, the two eyes and Outer *Laogong* (P. 8) at the back of the hand at the waist linear, as you exhale and inhale, the

small of your back fluctuates. Concentrate your attention on Inner *Laogong* (P. 8) of the raised hand when exhaling and on Outer *Laogong* (P. 8) of the lower hand when inhaling. The mind, the Inner *Laogong* (P. 8), the eyes and the small of the back should move slightly along with the fluctuation.

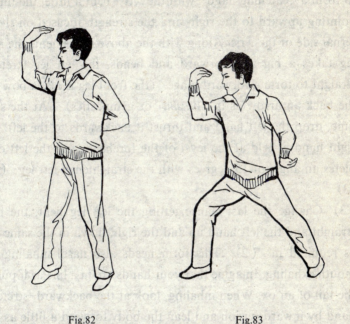

Fig.82   Fig.83

Form Five   Pulling Nine Oxen by Tails

1. Pityh Formula

   The front leg is a bow and the back an arrow;
   The lower abdomen is filled with *Qi* as if hollow.
   The strength is directed to the two arms,
   As if seizing something with the palms,
   And the eyes look inwardly at the hand they follow.

· 129 ·

2. Posture and Essentials
(1) Proceed from the last stance.
(2) Take the right hand off the right small of the back, drop it slightly, turn it naturally into *Yin* palm and thrust it forward until it is up to the shoulder level. Then bring the fingers together to form a "catching hand" with the wrist bent a little, the fingers pointing upward to the right and the strength focused on the internal side of the wrist. Along with the above movements, the right leg takes a big step forward and bends, the left leg stretches straight to form a forward lunge (the front leg is like a bow and the back an arrow as in *Wushu* or gymnastics). At the same time, drop the left hand and thrust it backwards to the left. The right hand is held at the level of the forehead, and the left completes an angle of 15 degrees with the straightened left leg (Fig. 83).
(3) Change the last stance, getting the left leg bent, the right straight and the left hand up and the right down in the same way as required in (2). This form needs also nasal inhaling and mouth exhaling. Imagine that your hands are in a line as if pulling the tail of an ox. When inhaling, look at the backward-stretched hand by inward-vision and lean the body forward a little as if to seize the tail, the forward and backward movement of the body being in coordination with the fluctuation of *Qi* in *Dantian* at the lower abdomen. The legs, waist, back, shoulders and the elbows, too, move or vibrate correspondingly to the forward-seizing and backward-pulling movement. Do this repeatedly for 3 – 5 times.

Form Six Stretching the Paws and Spreading the Wings
1. Pithy Formula

Stand erect and stare glaringly,
　　Push the window open to look at the moon steadily.
　　Topple the mountain and return the tide,
　　With respiration in guide,
　　And do it seven rounds straitly.
2. Posture and Essentials
(1) Proced from the last stance. Take the advantage of the "backward—pulling", get the bent leg back to stand with heels closed. Draw back the hands and hold them at the hypochondria, fingers straight upward and palms facing the front, to form "mountain—toppling palms".
(2) Push the "mountain—toppling palms" slowly forward. The forward pushing is very gentle as if pushing a window open. Stop the pushing when the shoulders, elbows and wrists are at the same level, then separate the fingers forcefully, keep the body straight, hold the breath, open the eyes widely, look straight ahead without any movement of the eyeballs or even a blink, and concentrate the mind on the palms (Fig. 84).
(3) Draw the "mountain—toppling palms" back slowly until they touch the hypochondria. Do the pushing and drawing for 7 times. Take nasal inhaling and mouth exhaling. Exhale when pushing gently forward, but hold breath somewhat when the arms are straight and begin to push with force to stretch the arms as much as possible as if gathering all the strength to topple a mountain. Exhale when drawing the palms back. Concentrate the attention on the two palms.

Form Seven　　Nine Ghosts Pulling Out Sabres
1. Pithy Formula
　　Turn the head and bend the elbow,

Hold the head and pull the ear,
Keep the right armpit open, And get the left closed.
Vibrate *Kunlun* with the right hand,
And touch the interscapular region with the left.
Change hands and repeat the same, With the body stretched and erect.

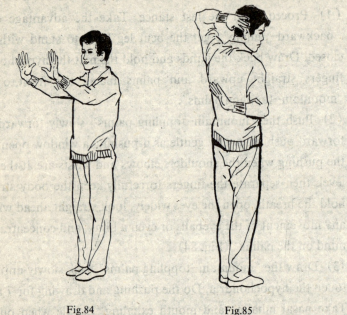

Fig.84 Fig.85

2. Posture and Essentials
(1) Proceed from the last stance.
(2) Raise the right hand to draw a semicircle towards the back of the head, apply the palm to *Yuzhenguan* (U.B. 9) at the occiput, press and pull the tip of the left ear (point *Tiancheng*, G.B. 9) with the index, middle and ring fingers, and keep the shoulder and the elbow parallel and the right armpit open. The

left hand draw half a circle leftwise until the back of the palm touch the interscapular region. Keep the left armpit closed tightly (Fig. 85).

(3) Let down the right hand and raise it backhanded to rest its back against the interscapular region. The left hand rises simultaneously at the back of the head, palm covering *Yuzhenguan* (G.B. 9) and the three fingers pressing and pulling the right ear gently with the left armpit open and the right closed tightly. This form needs nasal inspiration and mouth expiration. When inhaling, concentrate on the tip of the lifted elbow, which pulls upward a little, and move the head and neck in coordination with the manipulation of the hand. When exhaling, concentrate on the Outer *Laogong* (P. 8) at the back of the hand at the interscapular area and get *Qi* down to *Dantian*. Do the exercises 6 − 7 rounds.

Form Eight　　Three Dishes Falling to the Ground

1. Pithy Formula

　　The tongue is rested on the hard palate,
　　The eyes are open and the teeth gnashed,
　　The legs are bent in a horse—riding stance,
　　And the hands are pressing and holding;
　　The palms are turned and raised upwards,
　　As if a great amount of weight is added;
　　With mouth exhaling and nasal inhaling,
　　The feet are set firm and the body straight.

2. Posture and Essentials

(1) Proceed from the last stance. Raise and stretch out the arms sidewise to form a straight line at shoulder level, with the palms facing floor. At the same time, the left foot takes a big step to the

left to keep about 2.5 *Chi* (about 80cm) between the two feet (the distance can be altered according to the height of the individual practitioner).

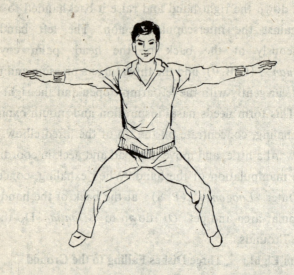

Fig.86

(2) Bend the knees and squat down slowly to form a horse stance, with the chest tucked in, the back straightened, and the angle between the thigh and shank being 90 degrees. Simultaneously, the two *Yin* palms press down until they are at the knee level (Fig. 86). The movement should be slow, and the strength exerted steady, with tongue stuck against the palate and eyes wide open.

(3) Turn palms up into *Yang* palms. Picturing holding something, move the palms upwards along with the straightening movement of the legs until they are at chest level. Do the exercise 3 — 5 times. Inhale by nose when straightening the legs and exhale by mouth when squatting down and let *Qi* down to

Dantian. Concentrate the mind on the two palms as if holding heavy things.

Form Nine   The Green Dragon Stretching Out Paws

1. Pithy Formula

  The green dragon stretches its paws,
  With the left one following the right.
  The left paw rolls and lowers, and tumbls and lowers,
  Below the ribs it stays.
  The right braves the wind forward,
  And the left "cloud gate" is exposed.
  Qi circulates around in the shoulders and back,
  And the waist and abdomen twisted.
  While uttering *"Xu"* gently to regulate breath,
  The movements of dragon and tiger are imitated.

2. Posture and Essentials

(1) Proceed from the last stance. Withdraw the left foot back to stand on feet shoulder-width apart.

(2) Turn the left palm to face floor to form a "dragon paw" (the joints of the fingers bent, the centre of the palm "empty" and round). By force of the waist, draw the left hand backwards with the tip of the elbow in the lead; at the same time turn the right palm to face floor and into "dragon paw", take advantage of the backward drawing of the left hand, stretch forward the right hand leftwise as if to brave the wind and the waves, to get the left *Qimen* (Liv.14) and *Yunmen* (Lu.4) points open and the right ones closed. As the left hand draws and the right stretches leftwise, turn the waist correspondingly and relax it as much as possible, by which the *Dai* Channel (Belt Channel) can be trained to be as flexible as silk and its tightness moderate (Fig.

87).

(3) Then withdraw the right hand and stretch the left rightwise in the same way mentioned above. Whichever hand is being stretched forward, you should utter "*Xu*" in cooperation and should turn the head and neck along with the movements of the hands. The exercise needs nasal inspiration and mouth expiration. Inhale during the process of withdrawing the left hand and stretching the right or vice versa and send *Qi* slowly down to *Dantian*; exhale when the withdrawing and stretching is done to the uttermost, while uttering "*Xu*", scratching gently for once with the third segments of the ten fingers and concentrating the mind on the two palms.

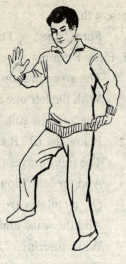

Fig.87

Form Ten   The Lying Tiger Pouncing on Its Prey

1. Pithy Formula

   Squat with feet apart to incline forward,
   Make the right leg an arrow and the left a bow.
   Hold up the head and chest to prostrate forward,
   Raise the hips towards the sky up and down.
   Inhale and exhale, the breath is evenly regulated,
   Touch the ground by fingertips in support.
   Lower the waist and back to flutuate,
   And withdraw the legs to resume upright standing.

2. Posture and Essentials

(1) Proceeding from the last stance, make a step forward to the

right with the right leg to make a forward lunge. Simultaneously stretch the hands forward to set the fingers on the ground, with the palms suspended (beginners may set the palms on the ground instead) and head raised slightly (Fig. 88).

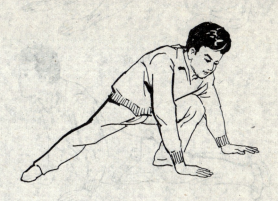

Fig.88

(2) Withdraw the right foot and rest its instep against the left heel. Do a push—up first and then lower the body and withdraw the buttocks slowly, with the eyes looking straight ahead, the waist relaxed as if a tiger ready to pounce on its prey (Fig.89).

(3) Hold up the head, prostrate the chest to about 4 *Cun* from the ground and get the head, waist, buttocks and extremities moving forward up and down like waves. Assuming a tiger ready to pounce on its prey, get the two eyes looking ahead and the waist relaxed. Throw out the chest a little when the arms are straight (Fig. 90), and tuck it in when the arms are bent. Do this for 3 — 5 times and return to the forward lunge.

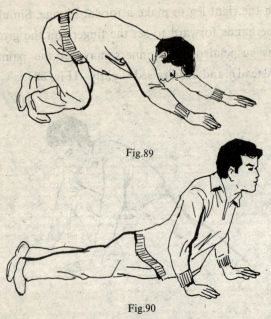

Fig.89

Fig.90

(4) Draw the right foot back to stand upright. The left foot takes a step forward to the left to make a forward lunge. Do right the same mentioned above for another 3 — 5 times. Return to the posture of the left forward lunge and then to the standing posture with feet shoulder—width apart.

The exercise requires nasal inspiration and mouth expiration. When the two palms are rested on the floor in a forward lunge, regulate the breath even. Inhale when the body is raised and exhale when it is lowered, with eyes looking forward as if going to pounce on something.

Form Eleven   Bending the Waist and Striking the Drum

1. Pithy Formula

   Hold the hind head with the palms and bend the waist low,
   Bring the head between the legs with teeth clenched and

mouth closed;
Rest the tongue gently on the palate and bend the elbows,
Cover the ears to strike the heavenly drums
As if an orchestra plays the eight tones.

2. Posture and Essentials

(1) Proceed from the last stance. Stand upright with feet apart as wide as the shoulders.

(2) Hold the head with both hands, palms covering the ears, the two middle fingers against *Yuzhenguan* (U.B. 9) with tips touching each other gently. The elbows are bent and raised to shoulder level. Strike with the two middle fingers at *Yuzhengua* (U.B. 9) repeatedly to give rub—a—dub in the ears. This is called "striking the heavenly drum" (Fig. 91).

(3) After striking, with hands still holding the head, bend slowly down as much as possible to get the head between the legs, with the legs straightened, the waist and buttocks relaxed, the tongue rested on the palate and the teeth clenched.

(4) Rise to get the body upright and beat the "heavenly drum" again and bend to repeat the above—mentioned for 3 — 5 times. Then return to the upright standing posture.

Take nasal respiration during the exercise. Hold breath slightly when bending down and rising (you can hold breath completely on rising after a period of practice). Concentrate the mind on *Dantian* when bending down and on the two palms when rising.

Form Twelve   Head and Tail Wagging

1. Pithy Formula

Straighten the knees, stretch the arms and
Push the palms to touch the ground,

Widely open the eyes, turn the head and
Focus the attention to be profound,
Erect the body, stamp the feet, strecth the arms and
Swag for 7 rounds,
And when this supurb exercise is practised,
Disease would be prevented and
Life would be prolonged.

2. Posture and Essentials

(1) Proceed from the last stance.
(2) Push the hands forward from the back of the head. Keep the arms stretched at shoulder level.
(3) Cross the ten fingers with palms facing floor. Withdraw the palms slowly towards the chest until they are two fists away from the chest, then push them downwards till the palms reach the floor with legs straightened. Push towards the middle, the left and the right once each, with the head nodding accordingly (Fig. 92) .
(4) Straighten the waist slowly to lift the palms. Let go the crossed fingers and wag left and right for 7 times each. Stamp the two feet alternately for 7 times at the same time.

Take natural respiration during practice. Keep the mind on the centre of the palms while you push the palms to the ground, and on the tip of the nose while standing straight.

Application

Sinew—transforming Exercise is aimed at building—up of the constitution.It is also a rudimentary exercise for emitting Qi (out—going Qi) . Practiced by young adults, it gives marketed results in keeping fit and disease prevention.

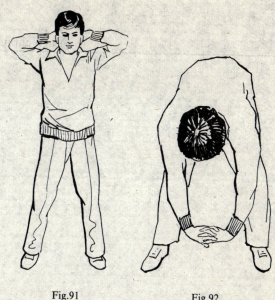

Fig.91　　　　Fig.92

Points for Attention

1. It is advisable to do the exercise once or twice a day.
2. Beginners should pay attention to adjustment of posture first, then to the coordination between breathing, mind activities and posture.
3. The old and middle-aged people should not let Qi go upwards during practice. The lifting of heels can be omitted, otherwise, rise of blood pressure, headache and dizziness may occur.
4. The exercise is one of the main dynamic exercises to train the skill of emitting out-going Qi.
5. The frequency of practice of each form should be decided flexibly according to the constitution and the health status of the

individuals, and it should be increased gradually. Never act with undue haste.

(Yu Wenping)

4 Emitting Out-going *Qi* (*Waiqi*)

4.1 Training of *Qi*

Training of *Qi* is the basic step of emitting *Qi*. A *Qigong* doctor usually has to undergo long-term physical (dynamic) and internal (static) exercises on posture, respiration and mind regulation before his functional activities of *Qi* can be voluntarily regulated, replenished and circulated down to Dantian, and his *Qi* can flow freely all over the body through the channels. Wherever his mind is concentrated, there is *Qi*; and wherever there is *Qi*, there is strength. This is the foundation for *Qigong* doctors to emit out-going *Qi*. Training of *Qi* is mainly achieved through static exercises, dynamic exercises and *Daoyin* selfmassage.

4.1.1 Static Exercise for Training *Qi*

(1) Posture

A sitting, standing or lying posture may be selected for the training of *Qi*. One may select the standing, upright sitting or the cross-legged sitting that is most suitable for him as the main posture and take the other standing and sitting positions as well as the lying posture as the supplementary ones so that he can take the advantage of any opportunities to practise. The essentials and methods of posture training are described in chapter 1.

(2) Respiration

Antidromic abdominal respiration is mainly adopted. The beginners may practice natural and then orthodromic abdominal respiration at the first stage, and when used to it, shift to antidromic respiration. The purpose for such respiration training is to get the breath deep, long, fine and even, the skill of which is nothing but a gradual accumulation of experience in respiration regulation. One cannot expect to master it overnight.

(3) Mind Regulation

Setting the mind on *Dantian* is the main method of mental concentration in training *Qi* in static *Qigong*. The method is literally called "concentration on *Qi* point", which is practised to gain substancialness of *Qi* in *Dantian* and to open the "small circulation" (*Xiao Zhou Tian*) or the "large circulation" (*Da Zhou Tian*).

(4) Methods

a. Be in a proper posture, relax all over and get rid of distractions. Imagine that the turbid *Qi* within the body is expelled through the mouth, nose and pores all over the body along with exhaling. After three times' exhaling, get the upper and lower teeth tapping each other for 36 times, then move the tongue within the mouth and swallow the saliva three times, imaging that the clear *Qi* of heaven and earth comes together with the saliva down to *Dantian* to nourish the whole body.

b. Both the regulation of smooth and even respiration and the concentration of mind on *Dantian* should be carried out naturally and lively. Voluntary holding of respiration and rigid mind concentration should be avoided. While you shoud not forget *Qi*, you should not speed up its circulation but simply follow it naturally as it progresses.

c. Training of *Qi* should be combined with nourishing of *Qi*. Conditions permitting, it is better to do *Qi* training sometime in the period from 11:00 p.m. to 1:00 a.m. and from 11:00 a.m. to 1:00 p.m.. During the rest of the day you can mainly practise nourishing of *Qi*. It goes without saying that in one episode of training, neither of the two aspects should be neglected. By the word training, it means that you should focus your attention, expel distractions and do the exercises by means of voluntary respiration and mind activities. The word nourishing here means your experience of a static inner health cultivation state, in which you present involuntary breathing and mind activities with the respiration soothing, relaxed, natural and soft and attention highly focused without any distracting. During the exercise, when you have entered "quiescence" by practising antidromic abdominal respiration and mind concentration on lower *Dantian* and you have achived relaxed body and soft, even and fine breathing, you can start to do inner health cultivation —— nourishing yourself. Only by combining training with nourishing, can you achieve satisfactory results.

d. This step can be called "*Qi* generating in *Dantian* and circulating all over". After a certain period of practice, *Qi* will be substantial in *Dantian* during exercising, and you may have a feeling of substantialness, warmth, or movement of *Qi* cluster or other strange but comfortable feeling. This sensation of *Qi* will become stronger and stronger as time goes by. When you have entered "quiescence", you may feel hot in *Dantian* and a stream of warm air (*Qi*) rushing from *Dantian* towards the coccyx area, which makes you relaxed and comfortable all over. Sometimes the point *Huiyin* (Ren 1) will throb first. Under this circumstance, you should guide genuine *Qi* to circulate along the *Du* Channel towards the two pairs of *Qigong* passes *Jiajiguan* and *Yuzhenguan* and further, through *Baihui* (Du 20) and go along the *Ren* Channel down back to *Dantian*. In this aspect, the principle of "focusing attention merely when *Qi* has not started to move and leading *Qi* to circulate when it is about to move" should be adhered to. To guide genuine *Qi* to flow in the *Ren* and *Du* Channels, mind concentration should be carried out in cooperation with breathing. When inhaling, conduct *Qi* to flow along the *Du* Channel to the Upper *Dantian*; when exhaling, conduct it to flow along the *Ren* Channel back to the Lower *Dantian*. This is traditionally called "small circulation" (*Xiao Zhou Tian*). As the time passes, when you get into the "quiescent" state, *Qi* gathered in *Dantian* will not disperse; it will circulate naturally along the *Ren* and *Du* Channels under the guidance of mind without the help of breathing.

e. Carry out the closing process seriously after each exercising session. This is the skill with which you may shift your mind slowly off the point you have been concentrating on, lead *Qi* to the Lower *Dantian*, relax yourself all over, open your eyes slowly, and do some selfmassage.

f. Selfmassage includes rubbing the hands, bathing the face (rubbing with palms), combing the hair with the fingertips and dredging the 12 channels. Rub from the chest to the hands to dredge the Three *Yang* Channels of Hand, and from the hands, the shoulders and the lateral sides of the head down to the chest and abdomen to dredge the Three *Yin* Channels of Hand. Rub from the waist and hips to the feet to dredge the Three *Yang* Channels of Foot, from the feet to the abdomen to dredge the Three *Yin* Channels of Foot. Repeat the above sequence 10 times. Limber yourself up to end the exercise.

4.1.2 Dynamic Exercise for Training *Qi*

Doing dynamic exercise to train *Qi* is to lay foundation for emission of out-gioing *Qi* in the field of *Daoyin* exercises. Static exercise is to gather *Qi* and to strengthen *Qi* internally, whereas dynamic exercise is to regulate the channels and to strengthen the bone and muscles (the physique) externally to ensure a free circulation of *Qi* so as to lay foundation for guiding *Qi*.

Sinew—Transforming Exercise
   (See 3.32 on page)

Double—nine *Yang* Exercise

This exercise should be practised on the basis of Sinew—Transforming Exercise. The practitioner first shakes his body in a spring vibration (like a pile being struck down) to make *Qi* in *Dantian* rippling. He also practises in a certain posture and with proper breathing and mind concentration to get *Qi* to circulate throughout the body. The exercise is to build up the physique and to activate the vitality of *Qi*. It is the foundational skill for mixed emission of *Qi*.

(1) Preparation
a. Basic Posture

   Take a standing posture as described below.

   Stand relaxed and quiet, with feet apart as wide as

shoulders, toes clutching at the ground, hands falling naturally, head picturing supporting an object on its top, eyes looking straight ahead but seeing nothing, tongue stuck against the palate, shoulders and elbows dropping, chest slightly out, buttocks slightly in, knees relaxed and bent somewhat, mind concentrated, and breath natural.

After adjustment of the posture, expel the turbid *Qi* three times along with exhaling as done in static *Qigong*. Then bend and stretch the knees alternately to cause *Dantian* and even the whole body to quiver and vibrate. The amplitude of vibration may be too large and unnatural at first. After some practice, however, the vibration will get easy and will converge towards *Dantian*, and eventually, occur with *Dantian* as the centre; the extremities will not vibrate or only vibrate slightly. This is a kind of pile—driving vibration —— vibration natural with small amplitude, which is required for all the exercise forms described hereafter.

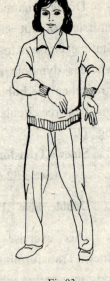

Fig.93

b. Massaging the *Dai* Channel (the Belt Channel)

Proceed from the last stance. Put the palms on the right side of the *Dai* Channel and massage it in cooperation with antidromic abdominal respiration. During inhaling, push the *Qi* of the *Dai* Channel with the palms (the right is preceded by the left) to flow leftwise, mind following palms to try to sense *Qi*, with the eyes slightly closed to get inward—vision on the *Dai*

Channel. During exhaling, push the *Qi* of the *Dai* Channel rightwise with the left palm preceded by the right in the same way mentioned above. Repeat the sequence for 9 respiratory cycles (Fig. 93). Carry out the same but with palms going rightwise when inhaling and leftwise when exhaling for another 9 respiratiry cycles to lead the flow of *Qi*

Breathing, posture and mind concenuration should be well coordinated during practice. The waist should be relaxed at the utmost and should rotate in small amplitude along with the motion of *Qi* induced by hand manipulations. You may feel your waist as soft as silk, the *Dai* Channel warm, the *Qi* flowing about the waist and circulating freely and vigorously all over the body.

c. Opening and Closing of the Three *Dantians*

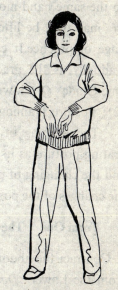

Take the standing pile—driving vibrating posture. When inhaling, get the back of the palms facing each other (the Outer *Laogong* pointing at each other) and then slowly get the hands apart at shoulders width. Meanwhile contract the abdomen and the anus, and get the *Qi* of nature into *Dantian*. When exhaling, get the Inner *Laogong* (P.8) facing the Lower

Fig.94

Dantian and draw the palms towards it slowly until they are one fist apart from it. At the same time bulge the abdomen and relax the anus and combine mind concentration, hand movement and *Dantian* in one. Gather the *Qi* you have sensed into *Dantian* and lead the *Qi* breathed in from the mouth and nose down to *Dantian* too. Repeat the above process for 9 respiratory cycles (Fig. 94).

Next, move the hands up to the level of the Middle *Dantian* (*Tanzhong*, Ren 17) and do the same open and close it for 9 respiratory cycles. Lifting *Qi* to the Middle *Dantian* while inhaling and sending the genuine *Qi* down to the Lower *Dantian* while exhaling.

The last step is to open and close the Upper *Dantian*. Move the hands up to the Upper *Dantian* (*Yintang*, Extra 1) and do the same hand movements for 9 respiratory cycles. However, *Qi* may only be lifted up to the Middle *Dantian* at the first stage of practice. It can be conducted to the Upper *Dantian* gradually as the practice is carried on for a longer period of time. Guide *Qi* down to the Lower *Dantian* during exhaling.

(2) Posture Training

The training of posture has the standing pile-driving vibrating posture as its basis, but one must combine the vibrating and the changing of posture in one to get *Qi* to flow following the changes of the posture.

Form One   The Immortals Pointing Out the Way

a. Contract the abdomen and anus during inhaling and lift *Qi* from the Lower *Dantian* up to the Middle *Dantian*, the two hands moving upwards simultaneously, palms facing upwards and elbows bent backwards, to the sides of the waist.

b. Exhaling, guide *Qi* to the right hand with the four fingers of the hand close together and the thumb stretched, the centre of the palm hollowed and the joint of the wrist bent up a little. By guiding *Qi*, direct internal strength to the arm, push the hand (palm erect) forward, and gather strength in the thenar eminance minor of the hand.

c. Inhaling, make fist and draw it back to the chest. Turn fist into palm facing downwards and press down. Turn the left palm up and lift it to hold *Qi* up to the Middle *Dantian*. Exhaling, push the left hand forward in the same method as described for the right hand. Repeat the process for 9 times for each hand. Finally get the hands back in front of the chest and hold *Qi* up to the Middle *Dantian*. Then get the palms facing each other to get prepared for the next step (Fig. 95).

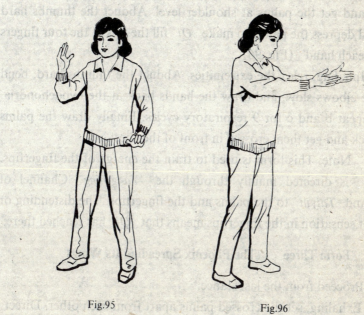

Fig.95   Fig.96

· 151 ·

Note: This form is used to train *Qi* of the *Shaoyin* and *Shaoyang* Channels. During expiration, direct the strength to the arm and push the hand out, with the palm dented a little to gather strength in it and then to the thenar eminance minor and further the small finger, i.e., to make *Qi* pass all through the Channels of Hand–*Shaoyin* and Hand–*Shaoyang*. Along with the vibrating *Qi* will be sent out from the Lower *Dantian* continuously and drawn back continuously into it.

Form Two   Pushing Eight Horses Forward

a. Proceed from the last stance
b. Exhaling, direct *Qi* to the shoulders and the arms. With the two palms facing each other, the thumbs stretched and the four fingers of each hand close to each other, push the hands out slowly and get the palms at shoulder level. Abduct the thumbs hard and depress the palms to make *Qi* fill the tips of the four fingers of each hand (Fig. 96).
c. Inhaling, relax the extremities. Abduct the thumbs hard, bend the elbows slow, and draw the hands back at the hypochondria. Repeat b and c for 9 respiratory cycles. Finally draw the palms back and get them crossed in front of the chest.

Note: This form is used to train the energy of the fingertips. *Qi* is directed mainly through the *Yangming* Channel of Hand–*Taiyin* to the palms and the fingertips. The distending or hot sensation in the fingertips means that *Qi* has reached there.

Form Three   The Phoenix Spreading Its Wings

a. Proceed from the last stance.
b. Exhaling, set the crossed palms apart from each other. Direct

Qi to the two arms, with the fingers bent back (the four fingers close together) as if the Inner *Laogong* (P. 8) was going to protrude. Get the back of the palms facing each other and push them apart until the hands, elbows and the shoulders are at the same level, with fingers still bent back and the Inner *Laogong* (P. 8) protruding (Fig. 97).

c. Inhaling, turn the palms so that they face each other, bend the elbows and draw the palms closer and closer to each other and finally get them crossed in front of the chest. Then draw them back to the sides of the chest to get prepared for the next step. Repeat b and c for 9 respiratory cycles.

Note: This form is aimed at training of the Channels of Hand—*Jueyin* and Hand—*Shaoyang*. *Qi* is accumulated in the Inner *Laogong* (P. 8) when the hands are pushed out, in the Outer *Laogong* and then is sent back to *Dantian* when the hands are drawn back. As a result of persistent training of this form, the line of *Qi* will always be kept round the palms, the centre of it is between the Inner and Outer *Laogong*. It is a very important form for guiding and emitting out—going *Qi*.

Form Four   Holding the Sky with the Hands

a. Proceed from the last stance.

b. Exhaling, lift the palms slowly. When they get to the point *Lianquan* (Ren 23), turn them sidewise slowly as if to hold something. Continue to lift them until they are above the head, with the arms stretched and the fingertips of the two hands pointing each other about a fist apart. The fingers should be closed together with the thumbs abducted (Fig. 98).

c. Inhaling, rotate the wrists to get the fingertips pointing upward. Lower the hands with the Inner *Laogong* (P. 8) facing the *Ren* Channel. Repeat b and c for 9 respiratory cycles. Put the hands at the sides of the chest with palms facing upward in preparation for the next step.

Note: This form is aimed at training *Qi* of the Three *Yin* Channels of Hand. It can make *Qi* flow along the *Yin* Channels of Hand to the face of the palms, then along the *Yang* Channels of Hand downwards.

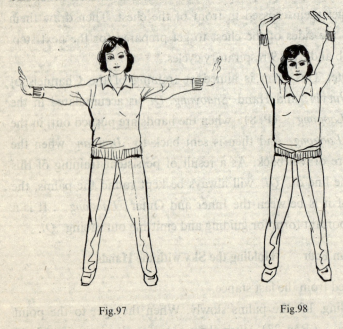

Fig.97　　　　　　　Fig.98

Form Five　　Scooping the Moon from Water

a. Proceed from the last stance.
b. Exhaling, get hands apart sidewise. Bend forward and hang down the arms, and draw hands between the feet with fingertips pointing at each other. until they are one fist apart. Accumulate

energy at the fingertips as if holding a bulky weight (Fig.99).

c. Inhaling, straighten the waist naturally to hold the "moon" up to the sides of the chest and direct *Qi* to *Dantian*. Repeat the above process for 9 respiratory cycles. Get the two palms upwards at the sides of the chest for the next step.

   Note: When bending forward, you should keep lithe and slow movement of your waist. The eyes are closed slightly to look at the "moon" (a round object or a light mass or a tiny glittering spot that can be taken as the moon) between your legs, and the hands probe, trying to catch the "moon" and then hold it up to *Dantian*. The exercise is good for nourishing *genuine Qi* and reinforcing the kidneys and can regulate both the *Ren* Channel and the *Du* Channel.

Form Six   Holding the Ball and Stroking It Three Times

a. Proceed from the last stance.

b. Exhaling, move the hands to the right side of the body with the palms facing each other, the left below the right, as if holding a ball. Inhaling, pull the palms a little farther away from each other as if the ball was being inflated and got bigger. Press the ball as if to compress the air inside it while exhaling. Repeat the above 3 respiratory cycles. Rotating the palms simultaneously, bring the right hand above the left to turn the "ball" upside down in front of the abdomen, and do the same "inflating" and "compressing" for 3 respiratory cycles there. Finally shift hands to the left side of the body and turn the "ball" upside down to get the left hand above the right, and do the "inflating" and "compressing" 3 respiratory cycles. Let hands stay at the left side for the next step(Fig.100).

Note: This form is practised for directing *Qi* (energy) to the palms and make it fill the six channels —— the Three *Yang* and Three *Yin* Channels of Hand. It is the art to guide *Qi* to circulate between the two palms by "holding a ball" with them.

Form Seven   Moving the Palms As If Setting Tiles on the Roof

a. Proceed from the last pose.

b. Inhaling, stretch the left palm forward and draw the right backward and vice versa when exhaling, to guide *Qi* of the Three *Yin* Channels of Hand for 9 respiratory cycles (Fig. 101). Get the hands at the sides of the chest, palms upwards, to be prepared for the next step.

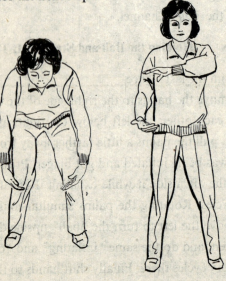

Fig.99   Fig.100

Note: This form is aimed at dredging the Three *Yin* and Three *Yang* Channels of Hand to get *Qi* to reach the palms.

Form Eight   The Wind Swaying the Lotus Leaf

a. Proceed from the last stance.

b. Exhaling, stretch out the palms slowly and get the palms and the elbows at shoulder level. Cross the palms with the left above the right, both still facing upward, to connect *Qi* of the *Yin* Channels of Hand with that of the *Yang*. Inhaling, depress the thenar eminence major a little to facilitate *Qi* along the channel of Hand–*Taiyin* to reach there and further to reach the tips of the thumbs. When exhaling again, stick up the thenar eminence minor to facilitate *Qi* to flow along the Channel of Hand–*Taiyang* to the thenar and the little fingertips. When inhaling again, draw the hands back to the chest. Do the above for 9 or 18 respiratory cycles. Put the hands (palms upward) at the chest to get ready for the next form (Fig. 102).

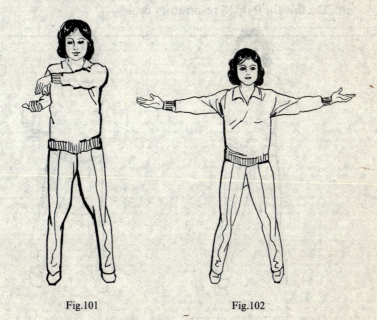

Fig.101   Fig.102

Note: This form activates the *Qi* of the Channels of Hand–*Taiyin*, Hand–*Taiyang*, Hand–*Shaoyin* and Hand–*Shaoyang*, making the *Qi* of *Taiyin* and *Taiyang* Channels circulate continuously.

Form Nine   Regulating *Qi* All Over

a. Proceed from the last stance.
b. Exhaling, turn the palms to get the fingertips pointing forward and stretch the palms out till the shoulders, elbows and wrists are at the same level (Fig. 103). Inhaling, turn the hands to get the back of the palms facing each other. Separate the palms to draw an arc with them and lift *Qi* to the armpits (Fig. 104), palms upwards and fingertips of the two hands pointing the sides of the chest. Stretch the palms out again when exhaling to draw another arc. Do this for 9 or 18 respiratory cycles.

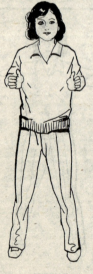
Fig.103

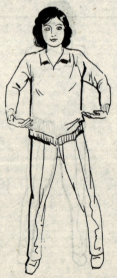
Fig.104

Note: This form is to combine the heavenly, earthly and human *Qi* in one as an organic whole and to regulate *Qi* of the whole body to get prepared for the closing of the exercise.

Closing Form of Double-Nine *Yang* Exercise:

Overlap the two hands with the right over the left (vice versa in female) and apply them to the Lower Dantian. Stop vibrating gradually and restore *Qi* into Dantian. Breathe naturally and concentrate on Dantian for a while. Rub your hands and face and move freely to end the exercise.

Kneading the Abdomen to Strengthen the Active Substance in the Body

The exercise is an auxiliary to static and dynamic *Qigong* in training *Qi*. The practice of it in combination with static and dynamic exercises can get the internal organs strengthened, intrinsic *Qi* reinforced, *Qi* accumulated without leaking, the strength multified, and the points opening and closing sensitively so that any risk of deviations can be avoided. This is especially important to those who carry out treatment of patients by emitting out-going *Qi* when they are versed in *Qigong* practice. If they do not practise this kind of exercises but treat patients, they may become insufficient in active substance, deficient in *Qi* and weak in strength. If they emit out-going *Qi* to treat patients, their health will be impaired easily by pathogenic *Qi* because they are not strong enough internally, their points are easy to open as soon as *Qi* reaches them and their resistance to external pathogenic factors is weak. This can cause local discomfort or morbid physical state which leads to a general disorder of *Qi* activities, resulting in collapse of the achievements gained through long-term practice. So Kneading the Abdomen to Strengthn the Active Substance is not only an auxilary exercise for strengthening the intrinsic *Qi*, but also an indispensable exercise for those who treat patients with out-going *Qi* to practise.

Methods

(1) Lie supine on the bed with both legs stretched naturally, hands at the sides of the body, the whole body (especially the vicera) relaxed, distracting thoughts expelled, breath natural, and tongue pressed against the palate.

(2) Apply the right palm (left palm for a female) to the abdomen under the xiphoid process and rotate the palm to knead the upper abdomen clockwise (for a female kneading with the left palm counterclockwise is tonifying as it is so for a male to knead with the right palm clockwise). Do not exert force intentionally lest the hand get stiff. The correct manipulation should be natural and gentle, which gives a soft sensation under the palm inside the upper abdomen. Avoid distractions. Keep inward-vision attentively and concentrate the mind on the Middle Dantian. One should neither forget the flowing of *Qi*, nor speed up its flow; just let it progress naturally. Maintain natural breath with a calm mind and try to get the pleasant feeling of warm, gentle and continuous flowing *Qi* under the palm. Each session of practice needs 15—30 minutes; the time can be increased gradually to one hour but overfatigue of the arm should be avoided. Carry out the kneading three times a day: in the morning, at noon and in the evening, or twice a day: in the morning and in the evening.

(3) After about a month's practice and as *Qi* accumulates gradually, you may feel that your stomach-*Qi* is consolidated and your appetite and sleep improved, and you may have "the

feeling of *Qi*" in the mid-upper abdomen when it is pressed. The straight muscles of the abdomen may have become more solid or bulged gradually, which may appear more apparently when you direct *Qi* or exert strength to it. At this stage, the midline from the xiphoid process to the navel may be still soft and dented, indicating that *Qi* in the *Ren* Channel (the Front Mid-line Channel) is still not substantial. To improve it, massage the midline with your palm root and strike along it gently with a "hollow" fist. The dent will disappear then, and *Qi* in *Ren* Channel is now rendered substantial. This usually takes one a hundred days to attain.

(4) As a following step, conduct kneading on the right side of the abdomen with the right palm first, in a way of spiral kneading from under the ribs down to the groin, for 12 times. Do the same with the left palm to the left abdomen counterclockwise for 12 times. Then massage with the right palm the lower abdomen where the Lower *Dantian* is located circularly for 15 – 30 minutes. Pat the same site with a "hollow fist" for some time after the massage. By so doing, *Dantian* and even the whole abdomen will become substantial with *Qi* and will be strong and solid in about a hundred days.

(5) The next step is to strike with a "hollow fist" on the mid-line of the chest and the right and left side of it, followed by massaging the Lower *Dantian* in the way mentioned in step 4. Long-term practice will make both the chest and the abdomen substantial with *Qi*, indicating that both the *Ren* and *Chong* Channels are full of *Qi*.

(6) At this stage, you can direct *Qi* into the *Du* Channel (the Back Mid-line Channel). Then, ask someone to pat along

your *Du* Channel and along the first and second collaterals of the Urinary Bladder Channel, up and down and vice versa alternately. Ask him to rub these places with his palm root in order to get *Qi* even and full. In this way, the *Du* Channel will be substantial with *Qi* in about a hundred days.

(7) When the *Ren* and *Du* Channels are filled with consolidated *Qi*, you can carry out patting yourself on the upper and lower extremities from above to below, with emphasis on the regions where there are plumpy muscles.

The patting or striking of other parts can be done either with the palm (fist) or a specially made wooden hammer.

With about one year's practice of the exercise Kneading the Abdomen to Strengthen the Active Substance in the Body, you may feel that you are full of substantial and vigorous *Qi* all over. Your resistance to external pathogenic factors will be strong, your points will be highly sensitive in opening and closing and will not be affected by turbid *Qi*. On this basis, you can take some time every day to do the kneading of the abdomen and patting on the extremities as a routine.

4.2 The Guiding of Qi

Guiding *Qi*, or directing *Qi*, means to guide intrinsic *Qi* to a certain part (a portion or a point of the hand, etc.) where out-going *Qi* is emitted. This is usually made only when one has undergone serious training of *Qi* and *Qi*-guiding exercises for long. On guiding *Qi*, one should have *Qi* follow the mind and should be able to control and feel the direction, pattern, nature and amount of intrinsic *Qi* as well as the direction it flows in. The exercise is aimed at laying solid foundations for hand—emitting of out—going *Qi*.

4.2.1 Standing Vibrating with Palms Closed to Guide *Qi*

(1) Posture

Take a standing pile—driving vibrating posture. Keep feet shoulder—width apart. Bend the arms to set the palms closed in front of the chest, fingertips pointing upward and elbows and wrists at the same level. Picture supporting an object on the head. Tuck in the chest and straighten the back. Relax the hips and knees. Rest the tongue on the palate. Close the eyes slightly (Fig. 105) .

(2) Guiding *Qi*

Breathe naturally and concentrate yourself on *Dantian*. When you feel the motion of *Qi* in *Dantian* (a sensation of warmth and *Qi* circulation) , have your mind follow *Qi* to go in the *Du* Channel and through the Three *Yang* Channels of Hand to the palms and the fingertips during exhaling; when inhaling, get *Qi* (with mind following it) back to *Dantian* along the same channels. When *Qi* is circulating freely, keep your attention on the palms and the fingertips with gentle natural breathing. You will feel your palms hot, the fingertips thicker, distending and tingling and vibrating slightly as if something were coming out of them.

(3) Practise the exercise once or twice a day, 5 − 10 minutes each time.

4.2.2 Single–finger Meditation to Guide *Qi*

(1) Posture

Take the stand pile–driving vibrating posture, the left hand lifted to the shoulder level, the wrist bent, the index finger straight and the rest curved, the tips of the thumb and the middle finger touching each other to form a ring; the right hand (in the same gesture as the left) is at the right side of the abdomen; the index fingers of the two hands pointing at each other (Fig. 106) .

(2) Guiding *Qi*

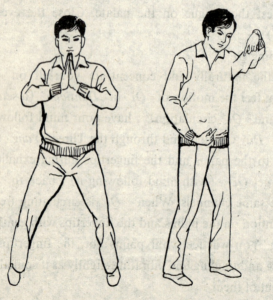

Fig.105   Fig.106

Breathe naturally and concentrate the attention on *Dantian*. As soon as *Qi* in *Dantian* is activated, begin to breathe slowly to direct *Qi* to the tip of the right index finger, and when you feel that *Qi* has reached there (you will feel your fingertip hot and distending as if something is being released from it), direct *Qi* from *Dantian* to the tip of the index finger of the left hand. As you feel that there is a tractive force between the tips of the two fingers caused by *Qi*, begin to rap with the tip of the left index finger on the *Qi* column being emitted from the right; you will get strong feeling of *Qi* at the two hands. Then direct *Qi* to the left index finger to emit it toward the right hand, driving the top of the *Qi* column to beat the tip of the right index finger; you will also get a strong feeling of *Qi*. Change your posture and the position of the two hands to train *Qi*.

(3) Do the exercise once or twice a day, 5 − 30 minutes each time.

4.2.3 Palm−pushing and Palm−pulling to Guide Qi

(1) Posture

Take the standing pile−driving vibrating posture. Release the fingers of both hands naturally. Stretch the right hand naturally forward to the right and bent the left to get it in front of the chest, the centre of the two palms facing each other. The same posture is assumed when the position of the two hands is exchanged (Fig. 107).

(2) Guiding *Qi*

Breathe naturally and concentrate the mind on *Dantian*. When *Qi* is activated, lead it to the Inner *Laogong* (P.8) of the left palm and emit it towards the Inner *Laogong* of the right palm. Push the palms toward each other while emitting *Qi*. Stop pushing to attract *Qi* between the palms, draw the palms back to the original position. You will get strong feeling of *Qi* when doing that. Exchange hands and carry out the same procedure.

(3) Do the exercise once or twice a day, 5 — 30 minutes each time.

4.2.4 Making Three Points Linear to Guide Qi

(1) Posture

Light a stick of sanitary incense. Put the incense burner on a table or you can take a similar object or a flower or a tree as a point. Take the standing pile—driving vibrating posture, the right palm stretched naturally in front of the incense, the burning tip of the incense pointing at the Inner *Laogong* (P. 8); the left palm, in the "single-finger-medication" gesture, put at the back of the tip of the burning incense, the fingertip pointing at the incense tip. The three points —— the left index fingertip, the tip of the burning incense and the Inner *Laogong* of the right palm are thus made linear (Fig. 108).

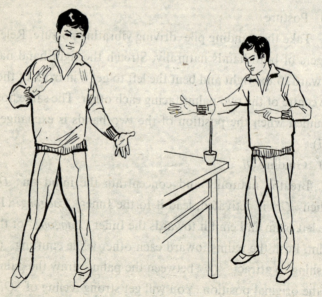

Fig.107　　　　　　　　Fig.108

(2) Guiding *Qi*

Proceed from the last stance. Breathe naturally and concentrate the attention on *Dantian*. When *Qi* in *Dantian* is activated, direct it to the tip of the left index finger. Exhale lightly and divert the attention onto the incense tip and concentrate there. Continue to emit *Qi* and send it farther on. You will have strong feeling of *Qi* in Inner *Laogong* of the right hand.

(3) Do the exercise once or twice a day, 5 – 30 minutes each time.

4.2.5 Making Three Points Circular to Guide Qi

(1) Posture

Stand vibrating. Burn a stick of sanitary incense and put the burner on a table, or you can take a similar object, a flower or a tree as a point. Stretch the two hands naturally, the three points —— the Inner *Laogong* of both hands and the tip of the burning incense forming an equilateral triangle. Draw a circle mentally based on the centre of the triangle and the three points. *Qi* will fill the circle when you guide it (Fig. 109).

(2) Guiding *Qi*

After you have drawn the circle mentally, get your breath natural and concentrate your attention on *Dantian*. When *Qi* in *Dantian* is activated, lead *Qi* to the Inner *Laogong* of both hands. Exhale lightly to emit *Qi* towards the incense tip so as to make the three points attract or support one another. Picture holding a ball with your hands. Move your hands in response to the sense of *Qi*; while one hand pulls, the other pushes or vice versa alternately.

(3) Do the exercise once or twice a day, 5 – 30 minutes each time.

4.2.6 Jumping to Guide Qi in Burst

(1) Posture

Stand with feet apart at shoulders width, bend the knees slowly, and make fists to gather *Qi*. Concentrate your attention on *Dantian* when inhaling; when exhaling, jump and suddenly stretch out of the hands from the front of the chest, fingers separated and palms facing forward, to present a gesture of "speading claws" (Fig. 110).

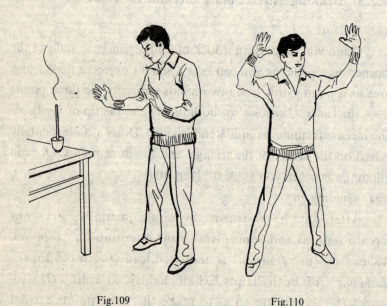

Fig.109　　　　　　　　Fig.110

(2) Guiding *Qi*

When inhaling, concentrate your attention on *Dantian*. Lift *Qi* to the chest and gather it in the palms. When exhaling, concentrate your attention on the centre of the palms with *Qi* bursting out from the Inner *Laogong* (P. 8).

(3) Do the exercise once or twice a day, 24 or 48 respiratory cycles each time.

4.2.7 Guiding *Qi* in Fixed Form

(1) Posture

Sit on or stand by the bed. Rest the left hand naturally on the left knee, put the right hand on the bed, the periphery of the palm touching the bed but the centre of it suspended, with the elbows bent a little, shoulders and elbows dropped and wrist relaxed.

(2) Guiding *Qi*

First of all, get the breath even and concentrate the attention on *Dantian*. When *Qi* in *Dantian* is activated, move the waist gently counterclockwise or clockwise. When inhaling, lift *Qi* to the chest, the intrinsic *Qi* vibrating and going upwards little by little from *Dantian* and finally reaching the palms on exhaling; and when exhaling, the vibration of the intrinsic *Qi* makes the palms to vibrate rhythmically, the frequency and force of the vibration changes with mind concentration. When *Qi* gets to the palm, it fills the palm and seethes there, you will feel as if there was an inflating ball under your hand. Yet *Qi* is always centred on the Inner *Laogong*, gathering together without dispersion. The motion of *Qi* and the movements of the hand are in perfect harmony.

The exercise is usually done in a sitting or a standing posture. The hand poses required for the training of guiding *Qi* in vibrational fixed form include middle-finger-propping (*Zhong*

Zhi Du Li Shi), spreading claw (*Tan Zhua Shi*), sword-thrust (*Jian Jue Shi*) and dragon-mouth (*Long Xian Shi*). When you can feel the vibration of the right hand, go on practising with one hand after another. After some practice of the exercise, you can come to train the *Qi* circulating form in different frequency, different intensity and different wave peak.

(3) Do the exercise 1 — 2 times a day, 30 — 60 minutes each time. Generally, the exercise can be preliminary mastered in three months.

4.2.8 Guiding Qi in Spiralty

(1) Posture

Any of the three postures (standing, sitting and lying) will do. The standing posture is taken hereof as an example.

Stand feet apart, place the right hand in front of the right side of the chest with the elbow bent, palm facing forward and fingertips pointing upward.

(2) On guiding *Qi*, get *Qi* in *Dantian* to turn inside the body counterclockwise in spiralty (*Qi* following mind concentration) through the chest and the upper extremities to the palms. Make *Qi* in *Dantian* to spiral (taking the navel as the centre) synchronously with that in the palms (taking the Inner *Laogong* as the centre). Beginners should do it slowly and increase the speed gradually and naturally. Don't be too anxious for quick results. The turning is flexible; you can turn from the smallest circle to the largest, or vice versa, or in other ways.

(3) The skill of guiding *Qi* described above can not be mastered overnight; you must do the exercise frequently, making full use of the standing, lying and sitting postures.

4.2.9 Cold and Heat Guidance of Qi

This form of *Qi*-guiding exercise conforms to the treatment principle of "treating the cold-syndrome with hot-natured drugs and heat-syndrome with cold-natured drugs".

Heat guidance of *Qi* needs, after adjustment of the posture, firstly to get the breath even and concentrate the mind on *Dantian*, imagining that the *Qi* in *Dantian* is as hot as a burning sun shining all over the body, and secondly to shift the hotness to the palms as if the hot sun was burning in and giving off heat from the palms or in and from the fingertips, or burning and giving off heat in other hand gestures.

Cold guidance of *Qi* should also begin with the regulation of even breathing and concentration of mind on *Dantian* and then on *Yongquan* (K. 1). Inhale the earthly *Qi* by way of heels and direct it to the chest and palms, imagining that the centre of the palm were as cold as ice, and concentrate the mind on the coldness there. Remember that you should not imagine that your whole body were such cold, nor should you direct such cold feeling to other locality lest it affect the coordination of *Qi* activities.

The exercise can be done together with other *Qi*-guiding exercises after you have mastered 4.2.1 and other exercises.

Of the above nine forms of exercises of quiding *Qi*, two or three can be selected for practice each time. After each session of practice, you should stand calmly for a moment, direct *Qi* back to *Dantian*, rub your hands and face and move about freely for a while to end the exercise.

4.3 Emission of Qi

Emission of *Qi* is also called "emitting method" (*Fa Gong*), "emitting of out-going *Qi*" (*Fafang Waiqi*), and in ancient times, "distributing *Qi*" (*Bu Qi*). It is a method adopted by those experienced in training *Qi* and guiding *Qi* who can direct their intrinsic *Qi* to the palms and fingertips or to a certain locality in other hand gestures, and emit it to the channels or points of the *Qi* recipient.

4.3.1 Hand Gestures for Emitting *Qi*

(1) Single-finger Meditation (*Yi Zhi Chan Shi*)

The index finger is stretched, the middle, ring and small bent naturally, the thumb bent gently over the back of the middle finger. Guide *Qi* to the tip of the index finger and emit *Qi* in touch of or off the part of the recipient being treated (Fig. 111).

(2) Flat-palm (*Ping Zhang Shi*)

The five fingers are stretched naturally. Direct *Qi* to the palm and, taking the Inner *Laogong* (P. 8) as the centre, emit *Qi* in touch of or off the part of the recipient being treated (Fig. 112).

(3) Spreading-claw (*Tan Zhua Shi*)

The five fingers are separated naturally, the finger joints bent to form a spreading-claw (as if to grasp something). Direct *Qi* to the fingertips and emit it in touch of or off the part of the recipient being treated (Fig. 113).

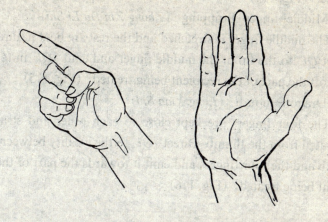

Fig.111   Fig.112

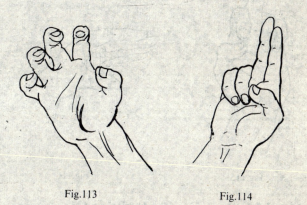

Fig.113   Fig.114

(4) Sword-thrust (*Jian Jue Shi*)

The index and middle fingers are kept close together, the ring and small fingers bent naturally and the thumb laid gently on their nails. Direct Qi to the tips of the index and middle fingers and emit *Qi* in touch of or off the part of the recipient being treated (Fig. 114).

(5) Middle-finger-Propping (*Zhong Zhi Du Li Shi*)

The middle finger is stretched and the rest are bent naturally. Direct *Qi* to the tip of the middle finger and emit *Qi* in touch of or off the part of the recipient being treated (Fig. 115).

(6) Dragon-mouth (*Long Xian Shi*)

The four fingers are kept close to each other and straight separated from the thumb. Direct *Qi* to the locality between the thumb and the four fingers and emit it towards the part of the recipient being treated (Fig. 116).

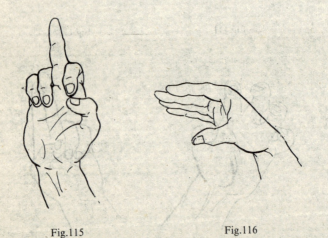

Fig.115 Fig.116

4.3.2 Hand Manipulations in Emitting Qi

(1) Manipulations with Hand Touching the Part Being Treated

a. Vibrating

Select a proper hand gesture. Lay the hand gently on the part to be treated and make vibrations to emit *Qi*. The method requires you to exert will to adjust the frequency, the amplitude, the nature and the amount of "*Li*" (power) and "*Qi*" (vital energy) during the emitting session.

b. Kneading

Select a proper hand gesture or use the tip of the thumb to conduct rotatory kneading with force on selected points or round the affected part, and simultaneously guide and emit *Qi*.

c. Rubbing

Select a proper hand gesture, or close the four fingers, to conduct rotatory massage slowly and forcefully on the select points, and at the same time guide and emit *Qi*.

d. Scrubbing

Scrub slowly with the flat palm or the flat of the four closed fingers in a straight line the affected part while guiding and emitting *Qi*.

e. Pressing

Select a proper hand gesture. Put the hand on the affected part. Exert press vertically while guiding and emitting *Qi*.

(2) Manipulations with Hand Off the Region Being Treated

a. Pushing

Select a proper hand gesture. Locate the hand about 15—100cm off the region to be treated. Guide *Qi* by making two point or three point linear or three-point circular. When you get the sensation of *Qi*, push your hand gently with "internal strength" to emit *Qi* to the region to be treated or to the related points.

b. Pulling

Select a proper hand gesture. Position the hand off the region to be treated. With the methods of making two point or three point linear or three point circular guide *Qi* slowly to the affected area or the related points. When you get the sensation of *Qi*, pull your hand gently with "internal strength" to emit *Qi* to the affected area.

c. Rotating

Select a proper hand gesture and keep the hand off the affected area, apply spiral *Qi*-guiding method to direct *Qi* slowly. When you get the sensation of *Qi*, conduct spiral hand manipulation clockwise or counterclockwise to guide *Qi* to flow in a spiral way and emit it into the affected area, or into the related points. You can also guide *Qi* slowly with the method of making three point circular to, and when you get the sensation of *Qi*, pull one hand and push the other gently and with "internal strength" to make circular motion to emit *Qi* to the affected area.

d. Guivering

Select a proper hand gesture and locate the hand off the region to be treated. Adopt the method "guiding *Qi* in fixed form" to guide *Qi* slowly. When you get the feeling of *Qi*, guiver the hand lightly to emit *Qi* fixedly to the region being treated or to the related points.

e. Leading

Select a proper hand posture and locate the hand off the diseased region to guide *Qi* slowly. When you get the sensation of *Qi*, emit *Qi* toward the affected area, and lead the channel *Qi* to flow with or against the run of the channels, leftwise or rightwise and upwards or downwards, depending on the severity of the illness.

f. Locating

Select a proper hand posture and locate the hand off the diseased region and guide Qi slowly. When you get the sensation of Qi, use one or several Qi— emitting methods to make fixed emission of Qi toward the region being treated.

(3) Auxiliary Manipulations

a. Tapping

Tap with one finger or the thumb and the index and middle fingers (closed together) along the channels or at the points.

b. Patting

Pat with the "empty" palm (fingers naturally stretched) on the disordered region, or along the channels, or on the points.

c. Hitting

Make a hollow fist and beat with its back or other parts on the disordered region, or along the channels, or on the points.

d. Pressing—intervally

Press intervally on the disordered region, or along the channels, or on the points with the tip of the thumb or the palm.

e. Stroking

Push and stroke with one palm or both palms along the channels or on the points or on the affected region.

f. Plucking

Pluck the selected points with the fingers.

g. Rubbing—to—and—fro

Press a certain part from both sides with the two palms or with the flat of the thumbs and the index and middle fingers. Rub the part to and fro gently, exerting force symmetrically.

h. Rocking

Rock or pull to and fro the joints of the extremities.

i. Rolling

Roll with the lateral side, near to the little finger, of the back of the hand on the region being treated, with the wrist joint bent and stretched and turned repeatedly.

4.3.3 The Forms of Qi on Emission

Clinical experience in emitting Qi has indicated that in treatment with out-going Qi, one of the keys to success is to emit Qi in different Qi forms according to needs. There are three basic Qi forms when it is emitted: linear, fixed and spiral. Having grasped the three forms, one can apply them flexibly in clinical treatment in agreement with the conditions of the illness and the changes of Qi, e.g., you may apply one form, or two forms in combination, or develop some special forms on the basis of the three. The application of the three basic forms can be put into pracitce in combination with the nature of Qi and the method of cold and heat guidance of Qi to form a combined Qi-guiding-emitting process.

(1) Linear Form

The "two-point line" method, "three-point line" method or other similar Qi- guiding methods are taken as the basic skills in training of the linear form Qi emission. Pushing, pulling, locating, leading and other hand manipulations are generally used to emit Qi. The linear form Qi emission is mild which gives a clear sensation of constriction, tugging, warmth and coldness. It is a basic form to induce channel Qi, supplement its deficiency and purge its excess. This form requires the hand manipulation in emitting Qi to be stable and slow, and the breathing to be deep and natural. It can also be carried out by means of deep and slow respiration.

(2) Fixed Form

This is a common Qi-emitting form with vibrating and fixed Qi-guiding method as the basic skills, and can be conducted with various hand manipulations. Emitting Qi this way gives marked stimulation to the activities of Qi in channels, points and Dantian. It is a major Qi form in mobilizing and stimulating Qi activities.

The method usually requires one to take an upright sitting posture or a horse-riding stance and natural and slow breathing. With the waist as the axle and the abdomen as the pump, make Qi inside the body vibrate and guide it to the part of the hand where it is emitted to the diseased part of the patient. The Qi is emitted like pearls, coming out one after another. The mind should follow the vibration of the Qi flow and give guidance to its flowing direction.

It merits special attention that when one carries out fixed emission of Qi, he must not hold his breath or make his hand vibrate by vibrating his muscles, otherwise stagnation of Qi will occur, resulting in stuffiness in the chest, pain in the hypochondria, sharp pain in the arms as if having a fracture, or laceration of the muscles.

To have a good grasp of this Qi-emiting method, one should first master the Qi-vibrating method to ensure that Qi is emitted naturally. Generally, one should carry out hand manipulation exercises in the order of training Qi, guiding Qi and vibrating Qi. A good grasp of the method of emitting Qi is no easy thing, for though one can expect to have a basic grasp of it in three months if he perseveres in doing the exercises, he can not expect to apply it skillfully to clinical treatment with only three months' practice.

(3) Spiral *Qi* Form

It is produced by the method "guiding *Qi* in spirality". *Qi* emitted this way goes spirally towards the affected area and penetrates deep. It provides special function in regulating *Qi* activities.

The emitting of *Qi* is induced by natural respiration and spiral mind concentration. The *Qi* starts whirling from the vortex in *Dantian* and moves in loops linked one with another to the part of the hand where it is emitted and where one can feel the whirling flow of *Qi*.

The learning of this skill needs not only constant practice of *Qi* rotation in *Dantian* but also the synchronized *Qi* rotation in a certain hand gesture. It is essential to form a fixed spiral *Qi*-flowing route so that when *Qi* in *Dantian* begins to rotate, it begins to whirl at the hand gesture simultaneously, and the flow of *Qi* can be regulated with the mind. Only then, can one start to apply the method to clinical treatment.

4.3.4 The Sensation of Qi

Sensation of *Qi* is actually the response to *Qi* by both *Qigong* doctors and patients during *Qigong* treatment. A *Qigong* doctor can diagnose the disease of the patient and adjust the procedures of treatment according to his feeling as well as the patient's feeling of *Qi*.

(1) The Sensation of Genuine *Qi*

The message of genuine *Qi* is often manifested as a slightly warm, cold, tingling, constricting or dragging sensation, or that of the flow of *Qi*. In most cases, the direction, density, nature and volume of the genuine *Qi* can be sensed.

(2) The Sensation of Filthy *Qi*

The sensation of filthy *Qi* is otherwise named "pathogenic message", which is different from pathogenic factors of infectious disease in modern medicine. Pathogenic message in *Qigong* can be classified as:

a. Cold Feeling

The *Qi* felt is especially cold. It may be so cold that when one gets such feeling of *Qi*, his fingertips get cold immediately, the terminal blood vessels will contract rapidly, and the coldness will transmit from the fingertips upwards, causing shivering and contraction of the sweat pores. This will give one a particular feeling of cold and discomfort.

b. Feeling of Dryness—heat

The message of *Qi* reacts on the body or hands of the *Qigong* doctor who gets a feeling of dryness—heat which makes him fidgety as if he were near a fire and being scorched.

c. Feeling of Soreness and Numbness

When such feeling of *Qi* occurs, one will experience local numbness and discomfort.

d. Feeling of Filthy *Qi*

Such filthy *Qi* can be felt when the *Qigong* doctor is standing or sitting opposite the patient or when the doctor is emitting *Qi* towards the patient. It gives the *Qigong* doctor an unbearable offensive feeling.

e. Other Kinds of Feeling

It has been said since the ancient times that there exist five kinds of pathogenic *Qi* such as joy and sorrow, and six pathogenic factors of excessiveness. Sometimes pathogenic *Qi* of joy can also be perceived if the *Qigong* doctor is quite attentive.

4.3.5 The Effect of Qi

When *Qigong* doctors emit *Qi* to treat patients, most of the patients may get some effect of *Qi* manifested as follows.

(1) The Phenomenon of *Qi*-sensitive Effect

When a *Qigong* doctor emits *Qi*, some patients may immediately or gradually get a feeling of *Qi* similar to or same as that occurring during *Qigong* practice, such as cold, hot, depressing, towing, creeping, tingling, heavy, light, floating and sinking. This represents a kind of *Qi*-sensitive effect occurring when *Qi* circulates in the channels and acts on the affected area to reach the focus. The most commomly felt sensation of *Qi* are cold, tingling, hot, depressing and towing.

(2) The Phenomenon of Dynamic Effect

When the doctor emits *Qi*, the patient may immediately or gradually show dynamic phenomenon —— involuntary movement of a certain part of the extremities or of the whole body. Some patients may have mild muscular tremor and others may get movements of the extremities in large amplitude. The phenomenon is known as simultaneously moving *Qigong* activated and induced by out-going *Qi*.

(3) The Phenomenon of Photoelectric Effect

On receiving out-going *Qi*, some patients may get some photoelectric effect manifested by a sensation of electric shock in the extremities. Others, with their eyes closed mildly, may see photopictures of different shapes, most of which are circular, patchy or lightening-like.

(4) The Phenomenon of Sound Effect

Some patients may hear some kinds of sound when they receive out-going Qi, such as "$La-La$", "$Long-Long$" or "$Zhi-Zhi$".

(5) The Phenomenon of Smell Effect

Some patients may smell a special odor on receiving out-going Qi. The odor usually varies in different patients. It may be the fragrance of sandalwood or that of flowers.

(6) The Phenomenon of Syncope Induced by Qi

A few patients may sweat all over with faster heart rate as can be seen in fainting during acupuncture when they are under out-going Qi treatment or have received Qi while waiting for treatment. Some patients may get syncope as well although they may have no apparant sensation of Qi and dynamic phenomenon, and in some, the illness may improve markedly after they have been activated by Qi and experienced syncope. The *Qigong* doctor should make the patients lie supine when they faint and carry out digital tapping on *Baihui* (Du 20), *Mingmen* (Du 4), *Jianjing* (G.B. 21) and *Yintang* (Extra 1), and grasping manipulation on *Jianjing* (G.B. 21), followed by conducting Qi along the *Ren* and *Du* Channels back to its origin. The patients can recover quickly this way.

The above-mentioned are the common phenomena of Qi effect, of which "phenomenon of Qi -sensitive effect" occurs most frequently, "dynamic phenomenon" occurs in a few patients and other phenomena occur very rarely.

The phenomenon of effect of Qi represents a special state of the sense and motion organs of the patients who have received out-going Qi from the doctors. It is rather a factor that decides the sensitivity of a certain sense organ and the channels of the patient than the pure therapeutic effect produced by *Qi* working on the diseased site. Some patients may show no apparant effect of *Qi* but recover very quickly after several courses of treatment and gain sensation of *Qi* gradually. Some may have no marked therapeutic effect though they show strong *Qi* effect. This is indeed a rather complicated problem which awaits further studies.

4.3.6 The Closing Form of Emission of *Qi*

(1) The Closing Form for Patients

When the *Qigong* doctor emits *Qi* to the patient, the patient will respond unvoluntarily as if he himself were doing the exercises. So when the treatment is over, the doctor should get the patient relaxed by restoring the patient's *Qi* back to its origin by means of hand manipulations such as digital tapping, patting, percussing, rubbing-to-and-fro and rocking, as the condition of the patient requires.

(2) The Closing Form for *Qigong* Doctors

To stop emitting *Qi*, the *Qigong* doctor should direct his *Qi* slowly back to *Dantian* and draw his hands off the *Qi*-emitting gesture. He should then readjust his mind, breathing and posture properly, relax all over and get genuine *Qi* back to its origin. If he is affected by pathogenic *Qi*, he should first expel it and then carry out the readjustment.

(Yu Wenping)

5 Treatment

5.1 Deviation of *Qigong*

Deviation of *Qigong* refers to the adverse reactions in the course of *Qigong* exercise. The practitioner feels uncomfortable and unable to control and remove them. Such reactions are physically and mentally harmful. Common causes of deviation of *Qigong* may include:

1. Exercising or practising under the guidance of an inexperienced instructor or the one who has no access to TCM theories which leads to failure to follow the righ way, or trying blindly to practise some method of *Qigong* exercise.

2. Failure to obey the principle of "exercising in light of concrete conditions", for example, those who are not fit for the exercise of intrinsic *Qi* circulation force themselves to do it.

3. Hoping to experience the quick results, some people fail to respond to the tiding and *Qi* effect in the correct way. And those who are mentally weak may have too heavy a psychological burden in the course of *Qigong* practice so that they gradually fall into victims of deviation.

4. Some practitioners sometimes fail to master the principle and methods of the "three regulations",fail to exercise in accordance with the given guidance, or change their styles now and then. All these may get themselves confused mentally and physically.

5. Fright or irritation possibly received in the course of *Qigong*

exercise may cause the deviation.

6. The practitioners blindly or unmaturely guide the intrinsic *Qi* to circulate or force the intrinsic *Qi* to go out.

7. Some practitioners get confused with or suspicious of the normal tiding phenomena occurring in the course of *Qigong* exercise, or ask unqualified *Qigong* practitioners for out-going *Qi* treatment. These may trigger their own out-going *Qi* to flow uncontrolled.

5.1.1 Deranged Flow of *Qi*

Symptoms:

Qi may get deranged and out of self control during or after *Qigong* exercise, which usually gives rise to dizziness, vertigo, panic, chest distress, short breath, uncontrolled movement of the extremities, tremor of the body, or causes *Qi* to flow without cease along a certain channel or in a certain location, making the practitioner very uncomfortable. In most cases, the victims are able to tell the location and direction of *Qi* flow.

Treatment:

1. Self-treatment with *Qigong* Exercise

Stop the *Qigong* exercises which have caused the symptoms mentioned above, get rid of panic and calm down the mind, shift the attention to concious movements. Then, pat the locations where *Qi* flows and carry out selfmassage along route and direction of the following channels: the Three *Yin* Channels of Hand, the Three *Yin* Channels of Foot, the Three *Yang* Channels of Hand and the Three *Yang* Channels of Foot. However, if the symptoms are severe, the patient should see an experienced *Qigong* doctor.

2. Treatment with Out-going *Qi*
(1) Select points in the location and along the channels where functional activities of *Qi* have been in a state of disorder. "Flat-palm" or "sword-thrust" hand gestures and pushing, pulling and quivering manipulations are used to help normalize the functional activities of *Qi* along the disordered or related channels.
(2) After that, pushing manipulation is applied to regulate *Yin* and *Yang* and to guide *Qi* to a certain channel, to certain viscera or to *Dantian*.

5.1.2 Stagnation of *Qi* and Stasis of Blood

Symptoms:

During or after *Qigong* exercises, disorder of *Qi* may occur, which then causes *Qi* stagnation and blood stasis in a certain location accompanied by the symptoms of pain, heaviness, sore and distending sensation and sensation of compression. These symptoms can not disappear automatically and may become worse if not treated.

Treatment:

1. Self-treatment with *Qigong* Exercise
(1) Stop the *Qigong* exercises which have caused the above-mentioned symptoms.
(2) If you feels a compressing sensation on the head and severe headache, you may massage the points *Baihui* (Du 20) , *Fengfu* (G.B. 20) , *Tianmen*, *Kangong* and *Taiyang* (Extra 2); then pat and massage along the route and direction of the *Du* Channel and the *Ren* Channel; still then concentrate the mind on the points *Yongquan* (K.1) and *Dadun* (Liv.1)

and carry out Head—Face Exercise in coorperation.

(3) If you feel tightened and compressed on the forehead, you may first massage the points *Tianmen, Kangong* and *Taiyang* (Extra 2), then pat from *Baihui* (Du 20) of the *Du* Channel down to *Dantian* along the *Ren* Channel. This should be done for several times. Then conduct pushing—massage from *Baihui* (Du 20) to *Dantian* for several times. Carry out the procedures in coorperation with Head—Face Exercise and Neck Exercise.

(4) If you feel distending pains around the point *Dazhui* (Du 14) ,you may apply pushing manipulation on *Dazhui* (Du 14) and *Jizhong* (Du 6) , and pat downwards along the *Du* Channel for several times. The above—mentioned therapeutic method may be used for the treatment of *Qi* stagnation and blood stasis of any location. Administration of drugs dispersing in nature and treatment by out—going *Qi* guidance and by inducing *Qi* with acupuncture are all prohibited.

2. Treatment with Out—going *Qi*

(1) In accordance with corresponding channel point selection, select certain points in and around the location where *Qi* stagnation and blood stasis exist. Tap and knead the points digitally and push and stroke along the channel.

(2) Flat—palm hand gesture and manipulative procedures of pushing, pulling and quivering are used to emit *Qi* so as to induce channel *Qi*. This out—going *Qi* is applied along the channel route to guide and normalize the functional activities of *Qi* and to dredge the channels.

5.1.3 Leaking of Genuine Qi (Vital *Qi*)

Symptoms:

During or after *Qigong* exercise, you may feel leaking of *Qi* from the external genitals, anus and some points, which can not be controlled by youself. Leaking of genuine *Qi* may lead to wasting, weakness of the extremities, pale greyish and dark complexion, vexation, failure of mind concentration, hypomnesis, spontaneous perspiration, night sweat, seminal emission, insomnia and reluctance to speak or move.

Trertment:

1. Self Treatment with *Qigong* Exercise

(1) Stop the *Qigong* exercises which have caused the symptoms. The victims may exercise anus contracting, teeth tapping and saliva swallowing among other techniques. They may pat the *Ren* Channel, the *Du* Channel and all the twelve regular channels along the direction of their course to ensure a smooth flow of *Qi*.

(2) The following prescription may be given to conduct *Qi* back to its origin.

Rhizoma Rehmanniae Praeparata (*Shudi*)	30 grams
Fructus Corni (*Shanyurou*)	30 grams
Radix Ginseng (*Renshen*)	9 grams
Magnetitum (*Cishi*)	30 grams
Radix Achy ranthis Bidentatae (*Niuxi*)	18 grams
Cortex Cinnamomi (*Rougui*)	6 grams
Os Draconis Fossilia (*Shenlonggu*)	30 grams
Concha Ostreae (*Shengmuli*)	30 grams

    Cinnabaris (*Zhusha*)   1 gram (taken following its infusion)

    The above drugs, except Cinnabaris, are prepared as one decoction given by oral administration, 5 — 10 doses altogether.

2. Treatment with Out-going *Qi*

(1) Press and knead the following points: *Shenshu* (U.B. 23), *Mingmen* (Du 4), *Dantian* and *Guanyuan* (Ren 4).

(2) Flat-palm hand gesture with pushing-locating manipulation is used to emit *Qi* towards the point *Mingmen* (Du 4), then, pushing-guiding manipulation is used to break through the channel and guide *Qi* to its origin. If *Qi* leaks from the external genitals, anus or the point *Huiyin* (Ren 1), guide it to flow upward to the Middle *Dantian*. If *Qi* leaks from the sweat pores all over the body, close the pores (points) and guide it to flow back to the Urinary Bladder Channel and the Lung Channel. If *Qi* leaks from the nasal cavity, treatment with out-going *Qi* is mainly focused on dredging the Lung and the *Ren* Channels.

5.1.4 Mental Derangement

Symptoms:

    During *Qigong* exercises, a phenomenon of mental derangement, also called "being infatuated" (*Ru Mo*), may appear in some practitioners who have regarded the illusion emerging during or after *Qigong* exercise as true, and this often leads to mental derangement manifested as uncommunicative and eccentric in disposition, withered and dull in expression, idle in movement, and apathy and trance. Some even lose their confidence of living and want to commit suicide; others suffer from continuous auditory hallucination and visual hallucination which are similar to that seen in psychotics. These symptoms are summerized as ten devils in *Zhong Lu Chuan Dao Ji* (Works of Zhong and Lu's Taoist Doctrine), which are the devil of six thieves, devil of animals, devil of aristocracy, devil of six passions, devil of love, devil of adversity, devil of saints, devil of fight, devil of amusement with women and devil of sexuality.

Treatment:

1. Self Treatment with *Qigong* Exercise

(1) Stop the *Qigong* exercises that have caused the symptoms. Turn a deaf ear to the auditory hallucination and a blind eye to the visual hallucination. Pay no heed to any illusion. Let the illusion emerge and disappear spontaneously. If the symptoms are severe, go and see a doctor for comprehensive treatment to obtain a quick and better therapeutic effect.

(2) The following prescription, modified *Baihe Dihuang Tang*, may be described for treatment.

Bulbus Lilii (Baihe)	30 grams
Radix Rehmanniae (Shengdihuang)	30 grams
Concha Ostreae (Shengmuli)	30 grams
Magnetitum (Cishi)	30 grams
Radix Achyranthis Bidentatae (Niuxi)	15 grams
Radix Polygalae (Yuanzhi)	12 grame
Semen Ziziphi Spinosae (Chaozaoren)	9 grams
Cinnabaris (Zhusha)	1 gram (taken following its infusion)

These drugs, except Cinnabaris, are decocted for oral administration.

2. Treatment with Out-going *Qi*

(1) Open the point of the Eight Extra-channels in accordance with *Ling Gui Ba Fa* (the Eight Methods of Intelligent Turtle), a theory of point selection, and with the principle of "opening the points at a definite time".

(2) Press and knead the points *Baihui* (Du 20), *Dazhui* (Du 14), *Lingtai* (Du 14) and *Feishu* (U.B.13); then use the Flat-palm or Sword-thrust hand gestures and pushing-pulling-quivering manipulation to emit *Qi* and guide *Qi* to flow along the channel.

(3) Pinch *Baihui* (Du 20), *Yintang* (Exitra 1), *Shangen* (radix naxi), *Renzhong* (Du 26), *Tinggong* (S.I. 19), *Jiache* (St. 6), *Quchi* (L.I. 11), *Hegu* (L.I. 4), *Weizhong* (U.B. 40) and *Chengshan* (U.B. 57).

(4) Middle-finger-propping hand gesture and vibrating method are used to emit *Qi* toward *Jiuwei* (Ren 15) and *Zhongwan* (Ren 12) for a period of 18 normal respiration, then guide *Qi* to flow along the *Ren* Channel back to *Dantian*.

5.1.5 Management of Temporary Symptoms Emerging during Qigong Exercise

Some mild symptoms may emerge during the course of initial practice. These symptoms, usually resulting from incorrect method exercise, should not be regarded as deviations and are not difficult to deal with. Introdueed below are some common symptoms and their management methods.

Fullness of the Head and Headache:

The facts that the *Qigong* beginners have not mastered the practising method and are too nervous mentally, their facial muscles are not relaxed, or mind control is exerted too much, are often the causes. Treatment methods include relaxation of the mind and muscles in the head during *Qigong* practice, Head *Daoyin* Exercise, Psychosomatic Relaxtion Exercise and the exercise saying "*Xu*".

Choking Sensation in the Chest:

This symptom usually stems from erroneous exercise of breath-holding and breath-prolonging. " Massaging the chest and '*He*' *Qi*" (exhale in puff) ,"massaging the chest and '*Si*' *Qi*", Chest Exercise, or concentrating the mind on the point *Zusanli* (St. 36) may relieve the symptom.

Abdominal Distention and Myoceliagia:

The two symptoms usually occur in beginners of the exercise Abdominal Respiration who do the exercise too lastedly and too streneously at the very beginning. To allay it, pay attention to proper movement of the abdominal muscles, have reasonable time duration of each exercise session, and do abdominal *Daoyin* exercise.

Coldness of the Extremities:

This symptom is mostly due to the practitioners' excess of *Yin* and deficiency of *Yang*, or by incorrect *Qigong* practice in terms of time, position and direction and breathing method. If the learners' practice methods are correct, they may leave the symptom alone and, as their *Yang-Qi* recovers gradually, the symptom will disappear. If the symptom is caused merely by incorrect practice method, you should get the method correct and do the exercise "taking essence from the sun" for supplement.

5.2 Syncope

Syncope, also called faint, is a state of temporary loss of consciousness which is usually caused by temporary cerebral ischemia or temporary cerebral anoxia, and often evoked by mental excitement, fright, severe pain, long-time standing or sudden rise to the feet. Traditional Chinese medicine holds that syncope is caused by disorder of *Qi*, or by *Qi* deficiency and collapse, or by failure of lucid *Yang* to rise.

Symptoms:

The victim is usually weak, experiencing dizziness, blurred vision, short breath and sweating, followed by faint with pale face, cold limbs, low blood pressure, fine and rapid pulse, reduced pupils, etc. Heavy needling, heavy manipulation in massage or treatment with out-going *Qi* may also cause syncope.

Treatment:

1. Self Treatment with *Qigong* Exercise

When premonitory symptoms of syncope emerge, the following procedures may be applied.

(1) Lay supine with the head being slightly lowered. Unbutton the collar, relax the whole body and take a deep breath, and guide *Qi* by mind to flow into *Dantian*.

(2) Press with the thumb nail *Renzhong* (Du 26), *Neiguan*

(P.6) , and *Hegu* (L.I.4) .

(3) Stretch the arms naturally at both sides of the body, breathe naturally with the tongue rested against the palate. Relax locally in the order of the head, neck, upper limbs, chest and abdomen, back and waist and the lower limbs. Take a rest for a while after the relaxation exercise is done three times.

2. Treatment with Out-going *Qi*

(1) Lie supine. Relax the whole body, pinch and knead the points *Baihui* (Du 20), *Renzhong* (Du 26), *Neiguan*(P.6), *Hegu*(L.I.4) and *Taichong* (Liv.3) to invigorate the vital function, replenish *Qi* and restore consciousness.

(2) Flat-palm gesture and pushing-pulling manipulation are applied to emit *Qi* toward the Lower *Dantian*, the Middle *Dantian* and the Upper *Dantian* to activate the functional activities of *Qi*. Then, flat-palm gesture and pushing-leading manipulation are used to guide *Qi* to the Lower *Dantian* from the point *Baihui* (Du 20) and along the *Ren* Channel. Still then, dredge *Qi* to the lower limbs (including the feet). Carry out the above procedures for 3 − 7 times repeatedly.

(3) Push and stroke the upper and lower limbs along the Three *Yang* Channels of Hand and the Three *Yang* Channels of Foot (beginning from above to below) with the pushing-stroking hand manipulation for 3 times. This may regulate the functional activities of *Qi* and invigorate *Qi* flow and blood circulation.

5.3 Common Cold

Common cold, known as URI (upper respiratory infection), refers to inflammataion of the respiratory tract caused by viruses or bacteria. The disease often occurs on climate changes or decline of the body resistance. TCM regards the cause of the disease as invasion of wind-cold, wind-heat or seasonal pathogenic factors.

Symptoms:

Symptoms of the wind-cold type are headache, nasal obstruction with watery discharge, sneezing, chilliness, anhidrosis, cough with thin phlegm, soreness of the joints, thin white tongue coating, and superficial tense pulse. Symptoms of the wind-heat type are headache with fever or sweating, dry mouth and sore throat, yellow nasal discharge, yellow sticky phlegm, thin and yellowish tongue coating, and rapid superficial pulse.

Treatment:

1. Self Treatment with *Qigong* Exercise

(1) Take a sitting or lying posture. Pinch and knead *Yintang* (Extra 1), *Taiyang* (Extra 2), *Quchi* (L.I.11) and *Hegu* (L.I.4) with the thumb.

(2) Do the Head-Face Exercise, Nose-Teeth Exercise as well as the procedures "dredge *Fengchi* and *Tianzhu*" as described in the Neck Exercise.

(3) Finally, dredge the Three *Yang* Channels of Hand, the Three *Yin* Channels of Hand, the Three *Yang* Channels of Foot and the Three *Yin* Channels of Foot as described in Shoulder-Arm Exercise and Exercise of the Lower Limbs.

2. Treatment with Out-going *Qi*

(1) With the patient sitting, pinch and knead *Yintang* (Extra 2), *Kangong*, *Quchi* (L.I. 11) and *Hegu* (L.I. 4) to open up the points and normalize the functional activities of *Qi*. Assume the flat-palm gesture and pushing-pulling manipulation to emit *Qi* toward *Yintang* (Extra 1) and *Taiyang* (Extra 2). Then use pulling-guiding manipulation to guide *Qi* to flow downward along the *Ren* Channel and the Stomach Channel of Foot-*Yangming* to both feet, 3 – 7 times are sufficient for expelling the wind-cold or wind-heat out from the feet along the channels.

(2) Press and knead *Fengfu* (Du 16), *Dazhui* (Du 14), *Fengmen* (U.B. 12) and *Feishu* (U.b.13). Emit *Qi* toward *Dazhui* (Du 14), *Fengmen* (U.B.12) and *Feishu* with flat-palm gesture and pushing-pulling manipulation. Then guide *Qi* to flow downward along the Urinary Bladder Channel of Foot-*Taiyang* with pulling-guiding manipulation. Stop guiding when the functional activities of *Qi* get balanced.

(3) Lastly, press and knead *Fengchi* (G.B.20), *Dazhui* (Du 14), *Fengmen* (U.B.12), *Quchi* (L.I.11) and *Hegu* (L.I.4) as well as the two upper limbs.

5.4 Epigastralgia

Pain in the epigastrium is the main symptom, which is caused, as traditional Chinese medicine holds, by the hyperactive liver-*Qi* attacking the stomach, insufficiency of the spleen-*Yang*, stagnation of *Qi* and stasis of blood. In addition, improper diet, climate change and mental factors may also give rise to epigastralgia, the symptoms of which are similar to that of chronic gastritis, gastric ulcer and duodenal ulcer.

Symptoms:

Symptoms caused by hyperactive liver—*Qi* attacking the stomach are: pain and fullness in the gastric region, vomiting and sour regurgitation which gets worse when excited, taut pulse and white, thin tongue fur. Symptoms caused by insufficiency of the spleen—*Yang* include relief of pain by pressing and warming, poor appitite, flatulence, watery vomitus, watery stools, clear urine, aversion to cold, white, thin tongue fur and slow pulse. Symptoms of epigastralgia caused by *Qi* stagnation or blood stasis are: localized pain in the epigastrium and tenderness, mass in the abdomen or black stool, reddened tongue, and taut and hesitant pulse.

Treatment:

1. Self Treatment with *Qigong* Exercise

(1) Conduct Psychosomatic Relxation Exercise and Inner Health Cultivation Exercise.

(2) The method "rubbing *Zhong Wan* Area and 'Hu' *Qi*" and the manipulation procedures of "dredying the spleen and stomach" described in Spleen Regulation Exercise may be practised by the patients with hyperactive liver—*Qi* attacking the stomach and with *Qi* stagnation and blood stasis; while patients with insufficiency of spleen—*Yang* should conduct manipulations of "rubbing *zhongwan* Area and '*Hu*' *Qi*" as well as "dredying the spleen and stomach" described in the Spleen Regulation Exercise.

(3) Chest—Hypochondrium Exercise and Abdominal Exercise should be done in cooperation with the above.

2. Treatment with Out-going *Qi*

(1) The patient should lie supine, relax all over, get rid of distractions, get the breath even and, when exhaling, guide *Qi* with mind to flow towards the gastric area where pain exists.

(2) The doctor should knead the location of ileocecal junction with the right hand and press the point *Jiuwei* (Ren 15) with the middle finger of the left hand. Regulation manipulation is used here to break through the point *Lanmen* (ileocecal junction).

(3) The doctor, with a flam-palm gesture and vibrating manipulation, emits *Qi* towards the gastric area for a period of 14 normal respiration. Then, middle-finger-propping gesture with vibrating manipulation is used in emitting *Qi* towards the points *Zhongwan* (Ren 12) and *Qihai* (Ren 6). *Qi* emission lasts for 14 normal respiration. Still then, push, rub and knead the abdomen in accordance with "pushing the abdomen to separate *Yin* and *Yang*".

(4) Use the flat-palm gesture and pushing-vibrating manipulation to emit *Qi* towards the point *Zhongwan* (Ren 12) (hand off it). Qi emission lasts for a period of 14 normal respiration. Then, with pushing-leading manipulation, guide *Qi* to flow towards *Dantian* along the *Ren* Channel, or to flow downward along the Stomach Channel of Foot-*Yangming*. Stop exercising when functional activities of *Qi* get balanced.

(5) The patient lies prostrate. The doctor kneads the points of *Pishu* (U.B.20), *Weishu* (U.B.21), *Ganshu* (U.B.18) as well as the Urinary Bladder Channel and the *Du* Channel, and emit out-going *Qi*, with vibrating manipulation, on the points of *Pishu* (U.B.20) and *Weishu* (U.B.21) for a period of 14

normal respiration. Then flat–palm gesture and pulling–leading manipulation are used to guide *Qi* to flow downward along the Urinary Bladder Channel of Foot–*Taiyang*.

5.5 Appendicitis

Appendicitis is commonly caused by appendiclausis or bacterial infection. It is called *Changyong* (periappendicular abscess) in traditional Chinese medicine, which holds that the "abscess" is caused by food stagnation, disfunction of the stomach and intestines, accumulation of dampness and heat in the intestines and *Qi* stagnation and blood stasis due to improper diet, sudden changes of the environmental temperature and intense movement immediately after a big meal.

Symptoms:

Pain is firstly felt at the epigastrium or around the umbilicus, which shifts down to the right hypogastrium several hours later (pain shift is characteristic of appendicitis) . The pain is dull and lasting, characterized by paroxysmal aggravation and accompanied by nausea, vomiting, constipation, diarrhoea, tenderness and rebounding pain at McBurney's point. The body temperature is around 37.5℃, and rises with the progress of the disease. If the body temperature is relatively higher and the abdominal pain stops suddenly, appendiceal perforation may exist. This requires timely surgical operation.

Treatment:

1. Self Treatment with *Qigong* Exercise

(1) The patient should lie supine and carry out relaxation exercise, paying attention mainly to the relaxation of the abdomen

and the viscera.

(2) Practise Exercise of Automatic Circulation of *Qi* and guide *Qi* with mind to circulate counterclockwise in the abdomen for a period of 18 normal respiration.

(3) Exert Abdominal Exercise with light and gentle hand manipulation.

2. Treatment with Out-going *Qi*

(1) The patient should lie supine. The points *Tianshu*(St. 25), *Lanwei* (Extra 33), *Zusanli* (St. 36) and *Shangjuxu* (St. 37) are pressed and kneaded to make *Qi* flow and normalize the functional activities of *Qi*. With the flat palm pressing on the umbilicus and McBurney's point, the doctor then emits *Qi* with slightly quivering manipulation for a period of 28 normal respiration.

(2) With the hand off the abdomen, the doctor emits *Qi* toward McBurney's point for a period of 14 normal respiration (flat-palm hand gesture and pushing-pulling manipulation are applied in this case). Then, pulling-leading method is used to dispel the pathogenic factors. Still then the doctor uses the same manipulation to guide *Qi* to flow from the abdomen downward through the Stomach Channel of Foot-*Yangming* to the lower limbs for 3 – 7 times.

(3) The patient lies prostrate. The doctor presses and kneads the points *Pishu* (U.B.20), *Weishu* (U.B.21) and *Dachangshu* (U.B.25), then apply the pushing-pulling-quivering manipulation and flam-palm hand gesture to guide *Qi* to flow downward to the lower limbs for 3 – 7 times to get the functional activities of *Qi* balanced in the upper and lower parts of the body.

5.6 Disorders of the Biliary Tract

Disorders of the biliary tract mainly include cholecystitis, cholelithiasis and ascariasis of the biliary tract. Traditional Chinese medicine holds that the first two diseases belong to the category of "hypochondria pain" or "jaundice", while the last is called biliary ascariasis. These disorders are mainly caused by mental depression, excessive intake of fatty food, exopathogenic invasion, stagnation of gallbladder–Qi and failure of biliary dredge resulting from stagnation of dampness and heat and obstruction or accumulation of ascarids. Though causes and symptoms of these disorders are different, $Qigong$ exercises for them and treatment with out–going Qi are almost the same. That is why they are jointly introduced hereof as a whole.

Symptoms:

The onset of these disorders are usually acute, and pain is felt on the right upper abdomen and on the right hypochondrium. Other symptoms are nausea, vomiting, rigor, high fever, yellow stained skin and sclera, whitish–grey stool when the biliary tract is completely blocked, and tenderness of the gallbladder when breathing deeply. Patients with biliary ascariasis may feel severe colic or a tearing sensation below the xiphoid process. The pain is so severe that the patient is wet with sweat, accompanied by nausea and vomiting. If the ascarid has withdrawn from the biliary tract, the pain is relieved immediately but can recur intercurrently. If the ascarid has moved completely into the gallbladder, the pain becomes continuous and distending; jaundice, rigor and high fever may appear; tenderness on the right part of the xiphoid process may be felt upon deep pressing.

Treatment:

1. Self Treatment with *Qigong* Exercise

(1) Sitting or lying, the patient can conduct relaxation exercise first, with stress laid on the relaxation of the back, waist, chest and abdomen. Several times of such exercises are needed.

(2) As a second step, the patient may practise "rubbing the hypochondrium and '*Xu*' *Qi*" as well as "soothing the liver to guide *Qi*" as described in Liver Regulation Exercise.

(3) Lastly the patient should practise Chest—Hypochondrium Exercise and Abdominal Exercise.

2. Treatment with Out—going *Qi*

(1) With the patient in a sitting posture, press and knead the points *Pishu* (U.B. 20), *Weishu* (U.B.21), *Ganshu* (U.B. 18), *Danshu* (U.B. 19), *Dannang* (Extra 36, a point of tenderness 2 *Cun* below the point *Yanglingquan*, G.B. 34) and *Zusanli* (St.36). Stress is laid on the points of the right side.

(2) Emit *Qi* towards the points *Pishu* (U.B. 20), *Weishu* (U.B. 21), *Ganshu* (U.B. 18) and *Danshu* (U.B. 19) on the right side for a period of 28 normal respiration, then emit *Qi* towards the pain location at the front side for a period of 28 normal respiration. Flam—palm hand gesture and vibratng manipulation are applied in the above—cited treatment.

(3) Emit *Qi* towards the gallbladder area at the front side for a period of 24 normal respiration. This is done with a flat—palm hand gesture and pulling—quivering manipulation. Then, pulling—guiding manipulation is used to guide *Qi* to flow downward along the Gallbladder Channel and the Stomach Channel.This may dispel the gallbladder—*Qi,* regulate *Qi* by

relieving epigastric distention and regulating the stomach.
(4) Press the point *Danshu* (U.B. 19) on the right side for a period of 12 normal respiration. Press and knead downward along the Urinary Bladder Channel on the two sides of the back and waist for 3 times.

5.7　Hiccup

Hiccup is habitually called *"Da E Te"* (belch), usually caused by spasm of the diaphragm due to excessive intake of raw, cold or pungent food, dispareunia, and adverse rising of the stomach—Qi resulting from liver—Qi attacking the stomach.
Symptoms:
Hiccup is continuous, usually lasting several minutes or hours and then ceasing without treatment in the mild cases; while in the severe cases, it may last, days and nights, which seriously interferes with mealing and sleep, getting the patient in a state of utter exhaustion. If hiccup occurs at a time when the patient has been sick for some time or in a state of severe illness, it may be a sign of crisis which deserves special attention
Treatment:
1. Self Treatment with *Qigong* Exercise
(1) Facing south, the patient may sit or stand, keep the feet apart as wide as the shoulders and relax the whole body. Then with antidromic abdominal respiration, he should take a deep breath and guide Qi to flow downward to *Dantian* during expiration, and further guide Qi to flow down to the point *Dadun* (Liv. 1) for a period of 3 – 9 normal respiration.
(2) Practise Chest—Hypochondrium Exercise and "massaging

the hypochondrium and '*Xu* *Qi*" of the Liver Regulation Exercise.

2. Treatment with Out-going *Qi*

(1) The patient should sit or stand, face south, relax and take normal breath, while the doctor pinches the point *Zhongge* (at the end of the line between the first two segments of the middle finger of the thumb side), presses and kneads *Pishu* (U.B. 20), *Geshu* (U.B.17), *Tanzhong* (Ren 17), *Zhongfu* (Lu. 1) and *Yunmen* (Lu. 2).

(2) Flat-palm hand gesture and pushing-pulling-leading manipulation are applied to emit *Qi* towards *Tanzhong* (Ren 17) and then, guide *Qi* to flow down to the lower limbs along the Stomach Channel of Foot-*Yangming*, which helps regulate the functional activities of *Qi*. Still then, the doctor should again emit *Qi* towards the points *Pishu* (U.B. 20), *Weishu* (U.B. 21) and *Ganshu* (U.B. 17) on the back, and guide *Qi* to flow downward along the Urinary Bladder Channel of Foot-*Taiyang*. This may normalize the functional activities of *Qi*.

(3) If the patient has not got improved, the doctor may emit *Qi* again towards the point *Baihui* (Du 20) and guide *Qi* to flow to *Dantian* along the *Ren* Channel, which is called "guiding *Qi* to its origin". All this is done with the flat-palm gesture and pushing-pulling-leading manipulatiion.

5.8 Gastroptosia

Gastroptosia is a chronic disease, referring to the descent of the stomach which is lower than its normal position. It is usually caused by protracted decline of digestive function, general malfunction, malnutrition and weakness. Traditional Chinese medicine believes that it is caused by weakness of the spleen and the stomach, and sinking of *Qi* of the middle—*Jiao* (*Zhongjiao*).

Symptoms:

Gastroptosia is characterised by epigastric bloatedness or abdominal distention which becomes severe when the patient stands up or lifts things after meal, and gets alleviated when lies down. This main symptom is often accompanied with belching, regurgitation of gastric juice or vomiting, poor appetite and wasting. Barium meal examination of gastric-intestinal tract provides a definite diagnosis.

Treatment:

1. Self Treatment with *Qigong* Exercise

(1) Lie supine with the sacrococcygeal region elevated by 4 Chinese *Cun*, take antidromic abdominal respiration, and practise Health Promotion Exercise.

(2) Practise Nine-Turn Exercise for Longevity and Abdominal Exercise.

2. Treatment with Out-going *Qi*

(1) The patient lies supine. The doctor presses *Zhongwan* (Ren 12), *Tiwei* (4 *Cun* above the umbilicus), *Weishang* (Extra 14, 2 *Cun* above the umbilicus and 4 *Cun* lateral to it) and *Zusanli* (St.36).

(2) Middle-finger hand gesture and vibrating manipulation are applied to emit *Qi* towards each of the points of *Zhongwan* (Ren 12), *Weishang* (Extra 14) and *Tiwei* for a period of 14 normal respiration. Then the hand gesture is changed to that of

flat—palm to emit *Qi* (with the vibrating method and the hand pressing the area of the gastric cavity). The doctor emits *Qi* for a period of 14 normal respiration. At the same time, the patient should breathe in with mind control and breathe out without mind control.

(3) The doctor uses flat—palm gesture and pushing—leading manipulation to emit *Qi* towards *Dantian* for a period of 14 normal respiration, then guide *Qi* to flow to the area of gastric cavity and emit *Qi* for another 14 normal respiration.

(4) The doctor presses and kneads *Pishu* (U.B. 20) and *Weishu* (U.B. 21), and then applies flat—palm gesture and vibrating manipulation to emit *Qi* towards the above—mentioned two points for a period of 14 normal respiration, and normalizes the functional activities of the Urinary Bladder Channel with pushing—leading manipulation.

5.9 Diarrhoea

Diarrhoea implies frequent defecation and loose or watery stool. It does not refer to hematochezia or tenesmus. Improper diet and exopathogenic factors may cause gastrointestinal dysfunction which results in diarrhoea. The disease is most prevalent in summer and autumn when dampness and heat, the two exopathogenic factors, are rampant. Deficiency of the spleen—*Yang* and the kidney—*Yang*, the internal pathogenic factor, may also cause chronic diarrhoea. An old saying holds that deficiency of the kidney makes frequent defecation and deficiency of the spleen impairs its function.

Symptoms:

Symptoms of diarrhoea may, in accordance with its causes and characteristics, be classified into three types —— diarrhoea due to cold, diarrhoea due to heat, and diarrhoea before down. Patients with diarrhoea due to cold generally suffers from intestinal gurgling and abdominal pain, loose stool with indigested food, watery stool, frequent clear urination without thirst, and deep and slow pulse. This type of diarrhoea is mostly caused by cold and deficiency of the spleen. As for diarrhoea due to heat, the symptoms are stinking, yellow and loose stool, burning sensation around the anus, thirst, restlessness, dark urine, frequent urination, yellowish tongue fur, wiry and rapid pulse, and fever in most cases. It is often caused by summer heat attack. Diarrhoea at down is due to weakness of kidney—*Yang* which results in indigestion of food. The patient usually defecates (loose stool) 2 — 3 times every day before dawn.

Treatment:

1. Self Treatment with *Qigong* Exercise

(1) Practise Automatic *Qi* Circulation Exercise (counterclockwise only) supplemented with Abdominal Exercise.

(2) Patients with diarrhoea caused by cold and dampness may practise Filthy—Elimination Exercise, while patients with diarrhoea at dawn may practise "taking essence from the sun".

2. Treatment with Out—going *Qi*

(1) Carry out digital point pressing on *Pishu* (U.B. 20), *Weishu* (U.B. 21) and *Dachangshu* (U.B. 25) to open through the *Shu* points (stream points). Then press, with the tip of the middle finger of the right hand, the point *Lanmen* (ileocecal junction) while pressing the point *Jiuwei*

(Ren 15) with the tip of the middle finger of the left hand to help normalize the functional activities of *Qi* there.

(2) Apply flat—palm gesture and vibrating manipulation to emit *Qi* toward *Zhongwan* (Ren 12), *Tianshu* (St. 25), *Duqi* (the umbilicus) and *Guanyuan* (Ren 14) for a period of 14 normal respiration. Then massage the abdomen 36 times (It has an effect of tonifying if it is a deficiency syndrome and of purging if it is an excess one).

(3) Apply flat—palm gesture and pushing—pulling manipulation to emit *Qi* towards the abdomen and, at the same time, to guide *Qi* to rotate clockwise or counterclockwise, and then guide *Qi* to flow downward along the Stomach Channel.

(4) Push from the coccyx up to the seventh thoracic vertebra with flat palm. Press and knead the Urinary Bladder Channel (both sides) and the point *Zusanli* (St. 36).

(5) For patients with diarrhoea at down, flat—palm gesture and pushing—rotating manipulation are used to emit *Qi* towards *Mingmen* (Du. 4, gate of life) and *Dantian* for a period of 9 — 10 normal respiration. For patients with diarrhoea due to cold and dampness, or due to heat and dampness, flat—palm gesture and pulling—guiding manipulation are used to guide *Qi* to flow downward along the Stomach Channel and then to guide *Qi* to flow out of the body through the points *Zusanli* (St. 36) and *Jiexi* (St. 41), or through the toes.

5.10 Constipation

Constipation may be regarded as a single disease or as a complication of other diseases. Causes of contipation are usually classified into 6 types: deficiency, excess, wind, cold, Qi and heat. Deficiency implies *Yang* deficiency or *Yin* deficiency of the lower—*Jiao* (*Xia Jiao*). If deficiency of *Yang* occurs, *Yin—Qi* may stagnate and fail to circulate; if deficiency of *Yin* occurs, secretion of the body fluid may be out of order, giving rise to dryness in the intestines. Excess means excess syndrome of the stomach which causes constipation. Wind implies syndrome due to wind; rampancy of wind results in constipation. Cold implies the accumulation of pathogenic cold which impairs the functional activities of *Qi*. *Qi* implies the stagnation of *Qi*. And heat means that heat hinders the secretion of the body fluid. Each of the above—mentioned six types may cause constipation.

Symptoms:

Symptoms of constipation are usually dry and hard stool, prolonged duration of defecation, difficulty in defecation though the patient has strong desire to defecate, and defecation every 3 − 5 days, or even 6 − 7 days. Clear urine, dry stool and difficulty in defecation are usually found in patients with constipation due to cold and deficiency. Dark urine and preference for cold food are seen in patients with constipation due to excess and heat. Cough, difficulty in breathing, cold extremities, fullness and distention of the abdomen and difficulty in defecation are met in patients with constipation due to wind and cold. Belching, depression in the chest and abdomen, fullness and distention in the chest and hypochondrium are found in patients with constipation due to *Qi* stagnation.

Treatment:

1. Self Treatment with *Qigong* Exercise

(1) Practise Automatic *Qi* Circulation Exercise, mainly turning clockwise. Abdominal Exercise and Nine-Turn Exercise for Longevity are practised as supplement.

(2) Patients with constipation due to excess, heat, deficiency and cold should, in addition, practise "rubbing Zhongwan and '*Hu*' *Qi*" described in Spleen Regulation Exercise.

2. Treatment with Out-going *Qi*

(1) Press and knead *Dachangshu* (U.B. 25), *Shenshu* (U.B. 23) and the eight-*liao* points of *Shangliao* (U.B. 31), *Ciliao* (U.B.34), *Zhongliao* (U.B. 33) and *Xialiao* (U.B. 34) to break through the *Shu* points (stream points) .Then, push *Qijiegu* the seven-segment bone down 50 times.

(2) Break through the point *Lanmen* (Extra 33) with the thumbs and the middle fingers of both hands. Then, emit *Qi*, with flat-palm gesture and vibrating manipulation, towards the point *Zhongwan* (Ren 12) for a period of 14 normal respiration,and emit *Qi*,with the dragon-mouth hand gesture and pushing-rotating manipulation towards the point *Tianshu* (St. 25) for a period of 14 normal respiration. Still then, emit *Qi*,with the same gesture and manipulation, towards the point *Guanyuan* (Ren 4) for a period of 8 normal respiration, followed by guiding *Qi* to rotate clockwise.

(3) Emit *Qi* with the hands off the part to be treated for a period of 8 normal respiration (with flal-palm gesture and pushing-pulling-rotating manipulation), then guide *Qi* to rotate clockwise to get its functional activities normalized.

5.11 Hypochondriac Pain

The cause of hypochondriac pain was clearly explained in *Huang Di Nei Jing* (The Yellow Emperor's Canon of Internal Medicine) which says: "Pain occurs below the hypochondrium when pathogenic factors invade the liver". Though hypochondriac pain may be caused by *Qi* stagnation, accumulation and blockage, phlegm stasis, deficiency or excess, it is always related to the liver and is commonly seen in patients with hypactivity of liver—*Yang* or stagnation of the liver—*Qi*.

Symptoms:

Hypochodriac pain on one side is more often than that on both side. Severe pain, cough and difficulty in breathing are seen in patients with excess syndrome; hypochondriac pain on both sides, taut pulse, bitter mouth are found in patients with excessive fire in the liver; weak pulse, dry throat, poor appetite, dull pain or stinging pain are found in patients with deficiency syndrome, including insufficiency of *Yin* of the liver and the kidney, which is sometimes caused by mental depression or hemorrhage.

Treatment:

1. Self Treatment with *Qigong* Exercise

(1) "Massaging the hypochondrium and '*Xu*' *Qi*" of Liver Regulation Exercise is eligible for patients with excess syndrome; while "taking 'black' *Qi*", which is included in Kidney Regulation Exercises, is eligible for patients with deficiency syndrome. Chest — Hypochondrium Exercise should be added in cooperation.

(2) Practise Nine—Turn Exercise for Longevity.

2. Treatment with Out-going *Qi*

(1) Conduct digital tapping pressing and kneading on the points *Tanzhong* (Ren 17), *Qimen* (Liv. 14), *Zhangmen* (Liv. 13), *Ganshu* (U.B. 18), *Geshu* (U.B. 17), *Zhigou* (S.J. 6) and *Yanglingquan* (G.B. 34) to break through them and to promote the flow of *Qi* and the circulation of blood in the Liver Channel.

(2) Emit *Qi* with flat-palm gesture and pushing-pulling-leading manipulation towards the pain region for a period of 11 or 22 normal respiration, then guide *Qi,* with pulling-leading manipulation, to flow downward along the Liver Channel. Guide *Qi* to flow from right to left and from left to right if the functional activities of *Qi* are not balanced.

(3) Tap digitally the point *Guanyuan* (Ren 4) and knead the point *Shenshu* (U.B. 23), then emit *Qi,* with the flat-palm and quivering manipulation, towards the lower abdomen with the point *Guanyuan* (Ren 4) as the centre for a period of 8 or 16 normal respiratiom.

5.12 Bronchitis

Bronchitis is a disease of the respiratory tract, with cough as its main symptom. Acute bronchitis is caused by bacterial or viral infection or by irritation of protracted smoking, while chronic bronchitis by frequent attacks of acute bronchitis or other diseases. Traditional Chinese medicine holds that bronchitis is classified into cough, cough with dyspnea, and phlegm retention, and that it is often caused by pathogenic factors of wind-cold, wind-heat, or excess of phlegm-dampness.

Symptoms:

Acute bronchitis is often manifested as cough due to exopathy. The onset is acute with symptoms of infection of the upper respiratory tract such as nasal obstruction, itching throat and dry cough, accompanied by fear of cold, fever, headache and general malaise. The cough is paroxysmal, with thin or thick phlegm. The tongue fur is white and thin, and the pulse floating and tense. If pathogenic wind—cold is transmitted into the interior of the body and causes heat syndrome, symptoms and signs such as yellow tongue fur, thick or purulent phlegm, floating and rapid pusle or slippery and rapid pulse will occur.

Chronic bronchitis is usually manifested by cough due to internal injury. The cough is frequent, more frequent in fall and winter or when climate changes. It becomes severe early in the morning or at night fall. The patient may have abundant phlegm and slippery and greasy tongue fur. Slippery pulse indicats excess of phlegm—dampness mauifested as abundant expectoration, purulent phlegm and phlegm with blood Thin and rapid pulse indicates injury of the collateral branches of the Lung Channel by heat. If attaks of chronic bronchitis are too frequent and the disease gets lingering, pulmonary emphysema will develop.

Treatment:

1. Self Treatment with *Qigong* Exercise

(1) Practise "taking 'white' *Qi*" of the Lung Regulation Exercise if the patient is suffering from deficiency syndrome; practise "rubbing the chest and *Si Qi*" of the Lung Regulation Exercise if the patient is suffering from excess syndrome. Either type of patients should practise "rugulating the lung and guiding *Qi*" of the Lung Regulation Exercise as well as Chest—Hypochondrium Ex-

ercise.

(2) Patients suffering from acute bronchitis with the symptoms of exterior syndrome such as headache and aversion to cold may practise Nose—Teeth Exercise and Head—Face Exercise.

(3) Those with deficiency of the spleen—Qi and lung—Qi may practise "taking yellow Qi" included in the Spleen Regulation Exercise; those with deficiency of kidney—Qi may practise "taking black Qi" included in the Kidney Regulation Exercise. All these patients may practise Health Promotion Exercise.

2. Treatment with Out—going Qi

(1) Press and knead, with the patient sitting, the points of *Tanzhong* (Ren 17) and *Feishu* (U.B. 13). If the patient is affected by exopathogen, the points *Tianmen, Kangong, Taiyang* (Extra 2) and *Fengmen* (U.B. 12) should be massaged.

(2) Emit Qi, with flat—palm gesture and pushing—pulling—quivering manipulation, towards the points *Tanzhong* (Ren. 17) and *Feishu* (U.B.13) for a period of 6 or 12 normal respiration. Then guide the channel Qi to flow along the Lung Channel.

Emit Qi, with vibrating manipulation, towards the point *Zhongwan* (Ren 12) for a period of 14 normal respiration, then guide Qi, with flat—palm gesture and pushing—leading manipulation, to flow downward along the Stomach Channel.

(3) Emit Qi, with flat—palm gesture and pushing—pulling manipulation, towards the points *Zhongwan* (Ren 12) and *Qihai* (Ren 6) for the patient with deficiency of the lung—Qi and spleen—Qi for a period of 8 normal respiration, and then guide Qi to flow along the *Ren* Channel to its origin. If the

patient is one with deficiency of kidney—*Qi*, flat—palm gesture and pushing—pulling —leading manipulation are used to emit *Qi* towards *Dantian* and *Mingmen* (Du 4, gate of life), for a period of 8 normal respiration.

(4) If the patient is one with wind—cold syndrome due to exuberant exopathy, flat—palm gesture and pulling—leading manipulation are applied to emit *Qi* towards the point *Tanzhong* (Ren 17) and guide *Qi* to flow along the Lung Channel and out of the body through the fingertips.

5.13 Bronchial Asthma

Bronchial asthma is an allergic disease, usually characterized by repeated attacks and paroxysmal dyspnea with wheeze. Traditional Chinese medicine holds that the disease is caused by invasion of wind—cold, improper diet, mental depression, deficiency of the spleen and lung due to fatigue, accumulation of phlegm—dampness in the lung, impairment of the ventilating and dispersing functions of the lung, or slipperiness of primordial *Qi* of the lower part of the body and failure of the kidney in receiving *Qi* (deficiency of kidney—*Qi* may cause dyspnea).

Symptoms:

Bronchial asthma falls into two types: excess syndrome and deficiency syndrome. The former is manifested by acute onset, dyspnea which often makes the patient keep his mouth open and the shoulders raised to gasp for breath, fullness in the chest, wheezing, floating and tense pulse, and thin and white tongue fur; while the latter is characterized by shortness and rapidness of breath, severe wheezing upon movement, pale face, sweating,

cold extremities, light—red tongue, and thin and weak pulse.
Treatment:
1. Self Treatment with *Qigong* Exercise
(1) Practise Psychosomatic Relaxation Exercise, Inner Health Cultivation Exercise and Chest — Hypochondrium Exercise.
(2) Patients with excess syndrome of stagnation of phlegm—dampness should, in addition, practise "rubbing the chest and '*Si*' *Qi*" which is included in the Lung Regulation Exercise; patients with deficiency of spleen—*Qi* and lung—*Qi* should, in addition, practise "taking white *Qi*" and "taking yellow *Qi*" which are included in Lung Regulation Exercise and Spleen Regulation Exercise respectively; patients with failure of the kidney in receiving *Qi* and with sweating and shortness of breath should, in addition, practise "taking black *Qi*" included in Kidney Regulation Exercise.
(3) Iron Crotch Exercise (*Tiedang Gong*) may be practised to tonify the kidney, strengthen *Yang* and replenish primordial *Qi*.
2. Treatment with Out—going *Qi*
(1) Carry out digital tapping and kneading on the points *Dingchuan* (Extra 17), *Tiantu* (Ren 22), *Tanzhong* (Ren 17), *Guanyuan* (Ren 4), *Feishu* (U.B. 13), *Pishu* (U.B. 20) and *Shenshu* (U.B. 23).
(2) Emit *Qi*, with flat—palm gesture and vibrating manipulation, towards *Dingchuan* (Extra 17), *Feishu* (U.B. 13) and *Pishu* (U.B. 20) for a period of 14 or 28 normal respiration. Then, with the hands off the body surface, guide *Qi*, with pushing—pulling manipulation, to flow downward along the *Du* Channel to *Mingmen* (Du 4). Guide *Qi* this way for 3

— 7 times.

(3) Emit *Qi*, with the dragon—mouth or flat—palm gesture and pushing—pulling—quivering manipulation, towards *Tiantu* (Extra 17) and *Tanzhong* (Ren 17), then guide *Qi* to flow along the *Ren* Channel to Dantian. This may make the adversely ascending *Qi* descend.

(4) If the patient is one with kidney deficiency and insufficiency of the kidney—*Yang*, flat—palm gesture and pushing—pulling manipulation are used to emit *Qi* towards *Mingmen* (the gate of life), *Dantian* and *Shenshu* (U.B. 23) to strengthen the kidney—*Yang*. If the patient is one with phlegm accumulation and dampness due to hypofunction of the spleen, the point *Fenglong* (St.40) may be pressed and kneaded, and pulling—leading manipulation may be applied to emit *Qi* towards *Tanzhong* (Ren 17) and to guide *Qi* to flow to the Stomach Channel of Foot—*Yangming* so that the phlegm can be expelled out of the body along the Stomach Channel and through the point *Zusanli* (St. 36).

5.14 Palpitation

Palpitation refers to the abnormal heart beat (cardiac impulse) which can be felt by the patients. It is a common symptom of neurosis and heart diseases of various kinds. Traditional Chinese medicine holds that palpitation is actually an irritability caused by fright or insufficiency of *Qi* and blood that fails to nourish the heart.

Symptoms:

Palmus is the main symptom, sometimes accompanied by

chest distress, nausea and vomiting. Palpitation is paroxysmal, usually induced by mental irritation, overstrain and excessive drinking or smoking.

Treatment:

1. Self Treatment with *Qigong* Exercise

(1) Practise Health Promotion Exercise, Inner Health Cultivation Exercise and Chest—Hypochodrium Exercise.

(2) Patients with excess syndrome may practise "rubbing the chest and '*Ha' Qi*" and "regulating the heart and guiding *Qi*", which are included in Heart Regulation Exercise. Patients with deficiency syndrome may practise "taking red *Qi*" and "regulating the heart and guiding *Qi*" described in Heart Regulation Exercise. Nine—Turn Exercise for Longevity may be practised in cooperation. Patients with insufficiency of kidney—*Qi* may practise, as a supplement, "strengthening the kidney and guiding *Qi*" in Kidney Regulation Exercise.

2. Treatment with Out—going *Qi*

(1) Press and Knead *Xinshu* (U.B. 15), *Ganshu* (U.B. 18), *Tanzhong* (Ren 17), *Jiuwei* (Ren 15) and *Lanmen* (ileocecal junction) to get them open and their functional activities of *Qi* activated.

(2) Apply the middle—finger—propping or the sword—thrust gesture and vibrating manipulation to emit *Qi* towards each of the points of *Xinshu* (U.B. 15), *Ganshu* (U.B. 18) and *Tanzhong* (Ren 17) for a period of 8 normal respiration. Then guide *Qi* to flow to *Dantian*.

(3) Patient with fright or dysphoria may get treated with dragon—mouth hand gesture and vibrating manipulation. The doctor may emit *Qi* towards *Jingming* (U.B. 1), *Yintang*

(Extra 1) and *Baihui* (Du 20) for a period of 8 normal respiration each. Then, the doctor may continue to emit *Qi* with the hands off these points and guide *Qi* to flow downward with pulling—leading manipulation to ensure a smooth flow of *Qi*.

5.15 Seminal Emission

Seminal emission falls into two kinds: nocturnal emission and spermatorrhoea. Nocturnal emission is usually caused by excess of ministerial fire, exuberance of the heart—*Yang*, deficiency of kidney—*Yin*, overstain and breakdown of the normal physiological coordination between the heart and the kidney, while spermatorrhoea is caused by failure of the kidney in storing reproductive essence and incompetence of orifice for discharging seminal fluid.

Symptoms:

Nocturnal emission refers to ejaculation when dreaming. It occurs once every 5 − 6 nights or every 3 − 4 nights and is accompanied with the symptoms of dizziness, vertigo, fatigue and abdominal pain. Spermatorrhoea refers to ejaculation not related to dream; it may occur at any time or upon thinking of sexual activities. Patients with spermatorrhoea often have lassitude of the extremities and poor memory. the disease can last for years.

Treatment:

1. Self Treatment with *Qigong* Exercise

(1) Practise *Yang*—Recuperation Exercise or Vital Essence Recovering Exercise. Waist Exercise and Kidney Regulation Exercise may be practised as supplements.

(2) Practise the Exercise for Nourishing the Kidney for Rejuve-

nation and the *Yang*-Recuperation Exercise. Iron Crotch Exercise can also be selected for treatment.

2. Treatment with Out-going *Qi*

(1) Press and knead *Shenshu* (U.B. 23), *Xinshu* (U.B. 15), *Mingmen* (Du 4), *Guanyuan* (Ren 4), *Zhongji* (Ren 3) and *Sanyinjiao* (Sp. 6).

(2) Emit *Qi*, with flat-palm gesture and vibrating manipulation, towards *Zhongwan* (Ren 12), *Guanyuan* (Ren 4) and *Mingmen* (Du 4) for a period of 8 - 12 normal respiration. Again, emit *Qi*, with flat-palm gesture and pushing-pulling-quivering manipulation, towards *Dantian* and *Mingmen* (Du 4), and guide *Qi* to flow upwards along the *Du* Channel to *Baihui* (Du 20) and then guide it to flow forward along the *Ren* Channel to *Dantian*.

(3) Emit *Qi*, with flat-palm gesture and pushing-leading manipulation, towards *Baihui* (Du 20) for a period of 8 normal respiration, and then guide *Qi* to flow along the *Ren* Channel to *Dantian*.

5.16 Impotence

Impotence is a disease manifesting itself as failure of penis erection or softness of the erected penis. It is usually caused by masturbation in adolescence or intemperance in sexual life. Anxiety which impairs the reproductive essence, constraint, depression and kidney impairment by fright may also give rise to impotence.

Symptoms:

Failure of normal penis erection or softness of the erected penis which collapses quickly are the main symptoms. These symptoms may also be accompanied by lassitude in the loins and legs, dizziness, vertigo, listlessness, myasthenia of the limbs and hypomnesis.

Treatment:

1. Self Treatment with *Qigong* Exercise

(1) Practise mainly Iron Crotch Exercise in cooperation with Exercise for Nourishing the Kidney for Rejuvenation and Waist Exercise.

(2) Patients with insufficiency of kidney−*Qi* may also practise Kidney Regulation Exercise; patients with physical weakness may, in addition, practise Nine−Turn Exercise for Longevity, Inner Health Cultivation Exercise or Health Promotion Exercise; patients with listlessness may practise Head−Face Exercise as a supplement.

2. Treatment with Out−going *Qi*

(1) Press and knead *Shenshu* (U.B.23), *Mingmen*(Du 4), *Guanyuan* (Ren 4) and *Sanyinjiao* (Sp.6) .

(2) Emit *Qi* with flat−palm and vibrating manipulation towars *Guanyuan* (Ren 4) for 12 normal respiration, then with middle−finger−propping and vibrating manipulation towards *Zhongji* (Ren 3) for 12 normal respiration, followed by emitting *Qi* with flat−plam and pushing−pulling manipulation towards *Mingmen*(Du 4) for 24 normal respiration.

(3) Emit *Qi* with flat−palm and pushing−pulling−rotating−leading manipulation towards *Mingmen* (Du 4) and *Dantian* for 24 normal respiration and guide *Qi* to flow counterclockwise.

5.17 Dysmenorrhea

Dysmenorrhea is a disease characterized mainly by lower abdominal pain during menstruation, which is often related to mental stress during menstrual period, cold invasion or cold diet. Traditional Chinese medicine holds that it is caused by cold invasion, cold diet, anxiety, anger, emotional depression, and insufficiency of *Qi* and blood. Dysmenorrhea is classfied into two types ——that of excess type and that of deficiency type.

Symptoms:

Patients with dysmenorrhea of excess type have the symptoms of lower abdominal pain prior to menstruation or frequent lower abdominal pain, interior heat, dry mouth, dark violet menstrual blood, and advanced menstrual period and taut and rapid pulse in most cases. Patients with dysmenorrhea of deficiency type have the symptoms of lower abdominal pain after menstruation which can be alleviated by warming and hand-pressing, scanty and thin menstrual blood, delayed menstruation, aversion to cold and fine and slippery pulse.

Treatment:

1. Self Treatment with *Qigong* Exercise

(1) Practise Nourishing the Kidney for Rejuvenation cooperated by Abdominal Exercise and Waist Exercise.

(2) Practise Automatic *Qi* Circulation Exercise, with *Qi* mainly circulating clockwise in patient with excess syndrome, and counterclockwise in patients with deficiency syndrome.

(3) Delicate patients with deficiency of both kinds may, in addition, practise Health Promotion Exercise or Inner Health Culti-

vation Exercise.

2. Treatment with Out-going *Qi*

(1) Press and knead with the fingertips *Qihai* (Ren 6), *Guanyuan* (Ren 4), *Zhongwan* (Ren 12) and *Shenshu* (U.B. 23) to break through these points.

(2) Emit *Qi,* with flat-palm or middle-finger-propping gesture and vibrating manipulation, towards *Zhongwan* (Ren 12), *Qihai* (Ren 6) and *Guanyuan* (Ren 4). Then conducting rotating rubbing on the lower abdomen, which has the replenishing effect in cases with deficiency and purging effect in cases with excess. Still then, press and knead *Sanyinjiao* (Sp. 6), *Yinlingquan* (Sp.9) and *Taixi* (K 3).

(3) Emit *Qi* towards the Lower *Dantian* with flat-palm gesture and pushing-pulling-rotating manipulation, and guide *Qi* to whirl round the umbilicus clockwise for cases with deficiency syndrome while counterclockwise for cases with excess syndrome.

(4) Emit *Qi,* with flat-palm gesture and fixed quivering manipulation, towards *Mingmen* (Du 4), *Shenshu* (U.B. 23) and the sacral region, then guide *Qi* to flow downward along the Urinary Bladder Channel to normalize the flow of it.

5.18   Chronic Pelvic Inflammation

Chronic pelvic inflammation refers to the chronic inflammation of the uterus, ovary, oviduct and the connective tissues in the pelvic cavity. It often occurs in one or more organs and is seen in women in their middle age. Traditional Chinese medicine holds that this disease is caused by stagnation of damp-heat or cold—dampness in the pelvic cavity or uterus.

Symptoms:

Patients with chronic pelvic inflammation usually have the symptoms of pain in the lower abdomin, hypostatic distension, soreness in the lumbosacral portion, pain and distension that become worse during menstruation or after strain and increased amount of vaginal discharge. Headache, fever and aversion to cold, among others,are the symptoms seen in the acute phase. If it is caused by damp—heat stagnation, vaginal discharge is usually yellowish—red in colour and stinking in odour,and the pulse is often slippery and rapid and the tongue fur is yellowish and greasy. If it is caused by cold—dampness stagnation, vaginal discharge is white and as stenchful as rotten fish, the tongue fur is white and greasy, and the pulse is deep and slow, or taut and slippery.

Treatment:

1. Self Treatment with *Qigong* Exercise

(1) Practise Health Promotion Exercise, Exercise Automatic *Qi* Circulation Exercise and Abdominal Exercise.

(2) Patients with obvious cold—dampness syndrome or damp—heat syndrome may, in addition, practise Filth—Elimination Exercise, and "rubbing *Zhong Wan* (Ren 12) Area and '*Hu*' *Qi*" and "dredging the spleen and stomach *Qi*" which are included in the Spleen Regulation Exercise. Patients with lumber pain and discomfort may, in addition, practise Waist Exercise.

2. Treatment with Out—going *Qi*

(1) Press and knead *Zhongwan* (Ren 12), *Daimai* (G.B. 26), *Zhongji* (Ren 3),*Pishu* (U.B. 20), *Mingmen* (Du 4), *Shenshu* (U.B. 23) and *Sanyinjiao* (Sp. 6).

(2) Emit *Qi,* with middle—finger—propping gesture and vibrating manipulation,towards each of the points of *Zhongwan* (Ren 12) , *Qihai* (Ren 6) and *Zhongji* (Ren 3) for a period of 8 normal respiration. Then emit *Qi,* with flat—palm gesture and pushing—pulling—leading manipulation, towards *Dantian, Qihai* (Ren 6) *Zhongji* (Ren 3) and *Tianshu* (St. 25) . Still then, guide *Qi* to flow downward along the Stomach Channel until the functional activities of *Qi* get normalized.

(3) Emit *Qi*,with flat—palm gesture and pushing—pulling—quivering manipulation, towards *Mingmen* (Du 4) and *Shenshu* (U.B. 23) for a period of 8 normal respiration respectively. Then regulate the *Dai* Channel (the Belt Channel) to get the functional activities of *Qi* normalized.

5.19 Metroptosis

The morbid status of uterus prolapsing below the line of ischiac spine or prolapsing out of the vaginal orifice is called metroptosis. Too many births, postpartum disorders or other diseases may cause loosening of the uterine ligament, and when abdominal pressure is increased to some extent, uterus prolapses. According to TCM, metroptosis is called *"Yinting"* and is caused by disorder of the *Dai* Channel, sinking of *Qi* of the middle—*Jiao (Zhongjiao),* debility of the *Chong* Channel and the *Ren* Channel or downward flow of damp—heat.

Symptoms:

Prolapsing sensation is felt in the pubic area,which is usually accompanied by lumbago and the sensation of heaviness and straining in the lower abdomen. The body and cervix of the uterus may all prolapse out of vaginal orifice in severe cases. The uterus may contract back when lying supine and may prolapse when standing and walking.

Treatment:

1. Self Treatment with *Qigong* Exercise

(1) Practise the exercise of Inner Health Cultivation with a posture of lying supine and the buttocks elevated. Practise Abdominal Exercise and Waist Exercise (except downward-pushing) for cooperation.

(2) Practise Automatic *Qi* Circulation Exercise and "taking yellow *Qi*" of the Spleen Regulation Exercise. In addition, practise *Daoyin* Exercise for Activating *Ren* and *Du* Channels and *Daoyin* Exercise for Ascending and Deacending *Yin* and *Yang,* with emphasis laid on ascending.

2. Treatment with Out-going *Qi*

(1) Press and knead *Baihui* (Du 20), *Qihai* (Ren 6), *Guilai* (St. 29), *Pishu* (U.B.20) and *Shenshu* (U.B. 23).

(2) Flat-palm or middle-finger-propping gesture and shaking manipulation are used to emit *Qi* towards *Baihui* (Du 20) and *Qihai* (Ren 6) for 8 normal respiration each, and towards *Pishu* (U.B. 20) and *Shenshu* (U.B. 23) for 14 normal respiration each.

(3) Emit *Qi*, with flat-palm gesture and pushing-pulling-quivering manipulation, towards *Baihui* (Du 20), *Mingmen* (Du 4), *Pishu* (U.B. 20), *Shenshu* (U.B. 23) and *Qihai* (Ren 6), then guide *Qi* to flow to the Middle *Dantian* (the xiphoid), to render *Qi* ascending.

(4) Emit *Qi,* with flat-palm gesture and pushing-leading

manipulation, towards *Sanyinjiao* (Sp. 6) and guide *Qi* to flow to the Middle *Dantian* to get *Qi* normalized.

5.20 Acute Mastitis

Acute mastitis is also called inflammation of the mammary glands which, as traditional Chinese medicine holds, is caused by stagnation of *Qi* and stasis of blood resulting from stagnation of the liver—*Qi* or the gallbladder—*Qi* and excessiveness of toxic heat in the Stomach Channel. Milk stagnation in the mammary glands, which is caused by trauma or extrusion, may give rise to acute mastitis. Acute mastitis infected via baby's mouth is called *"Chuiru"* and commonly seen in women in their lactation.

Symptoms:

Local swelling, fever, pain or masses accompanied with general fever and chills, nausea and polydipsia appearing at the first stage, followed by pustulation later.

Treatment:

1. Self Treatment with *Qigong* Exercise

(1) Patients at the first stage of the disease without pustulation may knead the surrounding area of the swelling gently with the tips of the index, middle, ring and little fingers (close together) and practise Chest—Hypochondrium Exercise.

(2) Practise "rubbing the chest and '*Xu*' *Qi*" of Liver Regulation Exercise, and "rubbing the abdomen and '*Hu*' *Qi*" of Spleen Regulation Exercise.

2. Treatment with Out—going *Qi*

Treatment with out—going *Qi* is efficacious only at the first stage of the disease. Incision and drainage are needed if abscess develops.

(1) Press and knead *Tanzhong* (Ren 17), *Rugen* (St. 18), *Zhongfu* (Lu.1), *Ganshu* (U.B. 18) and *Weishu* (U.B. 21) to open through the points along the Liver Channel, Stomach Channel and the Lung Channel.

(2) Flat—palm gesture and vibrating manipulation are applied to emit *Qi*, with the point Inner *Laogong* facing the swollen masses, for a period of 48 normal respiration. Then, apply dragon—mouth hand gesture (with *Qi* directed to the space between the thumb and the fingers) and vibrating manipulation to emit *Qi* for a period of 24 normal respiration. Still then, flat—palm gesture and pushing—pulling—leading manipulation are used to emit *Qi* towards the point *Ruzhong* (St.17) and guide *Qi* to flow along the Stomach Channel to open through the channel and guide the stomach—*Qi* to flow downward and expel the pathogenic factors out of the body.

(3) Gently pinch and extrude the breast with the thumb, index finger and middle finger to extrude the stagnated milk. This should be done once a day.

5.21 Stiff—neck

Stiff—neck refers to the simple acute stiffness and pain of the neck, which causes cervical immobilization. It is often caused by improper sleeping posture, invasion of pathogenic wind—dampness or obstruction of channels and collaterals.

Symptoms:

It is usually noticed in the morning when the patient feels pain on one side of the neck, difficult in turning the head, and sometimes radiation of pain to the shoulder and back. Cervical muscles are in a spasmodic state and local tenderness is obvious, but no swelling and local heat is found.

Treatment:

1. Self Treatment with *Qigong* Exercise

   Practise Neck Exercise, Shoulder-Arm Exercise and Brocade Exercise in Six Forms.

2. Treatment with Out-going *Qi*

(1) Press and knead *Tianzhu* (St. 25) and the Urinary Bladder Channel on the two sides of the neck, then press and knead *Fengchi* (G.B. 20), *Fengfu* (Du 16), *Jianzhongshu* (S.I. 15), *Jianwaishu* (S.I. 4), *Quchi* (L.I. 11) and *Hegu* (L.I. 4). This may help open through the points and dredge the channels and collaterals.

(2) With flat-palm gesture and pushing-pulling-leading manipulation, emit *Qi* towards the painful area of the neck, guide *Qi* to flow downward along the Urinary Bladder Channel and also guide *Qi* to flow to the upper arms along the Small Intestine Channel. This may help dredge the channels and collaterals and regulate the functional activities of *Qi*.

(3) The method of oblique pulling of the neck is applied to help relieve regidity of the joints and to regulate the muscles.

5.22 Pain in the Waist and Lower Extremities

Pain in the waist and lower extremities is often caused by exopathy of wind-coldness, invasion of wind-dampness into the channels and collaterals due to sitting or lying on damp ground, internal injury caused by overstrain, dificiency and weakness of kidney—*Qi*, insufficiency of vital essence and energy or trauma. It is a syndrome similar to the symptoms of protrusion of intervertebral disc, sciatica, etc.

Symptoms:

Patients with pain in the waist and lower extremities of the wind—cold—damp type often have the symptoms of soreness of the waist, difficulty in waist movement, radiation of pain to legs or feet in severe cases, aggravation of pain in cloudy weather and local sensation of coldness. Patients with pain in the waist due to kidney deficiency have symptoms of protracted and dull pain, lassitude in loins and legs, listlessness, and rapid and fine pulse. Patients with pain in waist and lower extremities due to trauma usually have the symptoms of marked tenderness, mild swelling and radiate pain along the Gallbladder Channel of Foot—*Shaoyang* or the Urinary Bladder Channel of Foot—*Taiyang* downward.

Treatment:

1. Self Treatment with *Qigong* Exercise

(1) Practise Waist Exercise and Exercise of the Lower Extremeties.

(2) Practise Brocade Exercise in Six Forms and Sinew—Transforming Exercise after the symptoms have been alleviated. This may help the patients recover and prevent recurrence.

2. Treatment with Out—going *Qi*

(1) Press and knead *Shenshu* (U.B. 23), *Mingmen* (Du 4), *Yaoyangguan* (Du 3), *Huantiao* (G.B. 30), *Yanglingquan* (G.B. 34), *Weizhong* (U.B. 40), *Chengshan* (U.B. 57), *Kunlun* (U.B. 60) and *Taixi* (K 3). This is to dredge the channels and promote channel *Qi* to flow.

(2) Emit *Qi* towards *Mingmen* (Du 4) and *Shenshu* (U.B.23) with flat–palm gesture and pushing–pulling–leading manipulation, and guide *Qi* to flow downward along the Urinary Bladder Channel of Foot–*Taiyang*.

(3) With flat–palm gesture and pushing–pulling–leading manipulation, emit *Qi* towards *Huantiao* (G.B. 30) and guide *Qi* to flow towards the lower extremities along the Gall Bladder Channel of Foot–*Shaoyang* to help dredge the channel.

(4) Carry out oblique pulling of the waist, palm–patting and passive movements of waist, hips and knees to relieve rigidity of the joints, relax muscles and tendons and promote blood circulation.

5.23 Headache

Headache is a subjective symptom that can be found in many diseases, acute or chronic. Traditional Chinese medicine holds that headache is caused by internal injury or exopathy, e.g., invasion of exopathogenic wind–cold into the vertex and then into the brain via channels, adverse rising of the accumulated stomach–heat, insufficiency of *Qi* and blood, improper preservation of reservoir of marrow (refering to the brain), stagnation of phlegm–dampness, lucid *Yang* failing to rise, excessive fire of the liver and gallbladder, etc. Head is the pivot of all the *Yang* channels and collaterals, and channel–*Qi*, collateral–*Qi* and *Qi* of the viscera all meet in the head. So headache of various types are named after the routes of channels.

Symptoms:

(1) *Yangming* Headache (Sinciput Pain)

Pain in the forehead is most obvious because *Yangming* Channel goes to the forehead along the headline, accompanied by dry thirst, dysphoria with feverish sensation, foul breath, constipation, yellow tongue fur and forceful or slippery and rapid pulse.

(2) *Shaoyang* Headache (Migraine)

Pain in one side, sensation of excessive heat in head and splitting pain are the main symptoms which are often accompanied by conjunctival congestion, hypochondriac pain, bitter taste in the mouth, dry throat, yellow and dry tongue fur, and taut and rapid pusle.

(3) *Taiyang* Headache (Occipital Pain)

Pain in the occipito-posterior position is the main symptom which is accompanied by fever, aversion to cold, stiffness and pain in the neck and back, thin and white tongue fur, and floating and tense pulse.

(4) *Jueyin* Headache (Vertex Pain)

Because the Channels of Foot-*Jueyin* meet at the vertex, pain in the vertex is the main symptom which is accompanied by vertigo, vexation, quick temper, flushed face, bitter taste in the mouth, insomnia, reddened tongue with yellow fur, and taut and rapid or fine and rapid pulse.

Treatment:

1. Self Treatment with *Qigong* Exercise

(1) Practise Psychosomatic Relaxation Exercise, with emphasis put on relaxation of the channels related to the pain area, e.g., the Stomach Channel of Foot-*Yangming*, and the Large Intestine Channel of Hand-*Yangming* for *Yangming* headache; the Gall Bladder Channel of Foot-*Shaoyang* and the Tri-*Jiao*

(*Sanjiao*) Channel of Hand—*Shaoyang* for *Shaoyang* headache; Urinary Bladder Channel of Foot—*Taiyang* and the Small Intestine Channel of Hand—*Taiyang* for *Taiyang* headache; and the Liver Channel of Foot for *Jueyin* headache.

(2) Practise Head—Face Exercise, Nine—Turn Exercise for Longevity and Brocade Exercise in Six Forms.

2. Treatment with Out—going *Qi*

(1) Press and knead the following points according to the location of pain: *Yintang* (Extra 1), *Touwei* (St. 8), *Hegu* (L.I. 4) and *Zusanli* (St. 36) in case of *Yangming* headache; *Taiyang* (Extra 2), *Xuanlu* (G.B. 5) and *Yanglingquan* (G.B. 34) in case of *Shaoyang* headache; *Fengfu* (Du 16), *Fengchi* (G.B. 20), *Tianzhu* (U.B. 20), *Jianzhongshu* (S.I. 15), *Jianwaishu* (S.I. 14) and *Houxi* (S.I. 3) in case of *Taiyang* headache; *Baihui* (Du 20), *Yanglingquan* (G.B. 34) and *Taixi* (K. 3) in case of *Jueyin* headache.

(2) Emit *Qi* towards the pain area with flat—palm gesture and pushing—pulling—leading manipulation, and guide *Qi* downward from the head along the channels with pushing—leading manipulation.

To treat pain on one side of the head, emit *Qi* first towards the pain area to promote the functional activities of *Qi*, then guide *Qi* to flow to the fingertips along the Tri—*Jiao* Channel of Hand—*Shaoyang* with pulling—leading manipulation, still then, guide *Qi* to flow downward to the lower extremities along the Gall—Bladder Channel of Foot—*Shaoyang* with the same manipulation, so as to make the functional activities of *Qi* deficient in the upper and excessive in the lower, or balanced all over.

(3) Flat—palm gesture and pushing—pulling—rotating manipulation are used to emit Qi towards the lateral sides, the front and the back of the head to normalize the functional activities of Qi.

5.24　Insomnia

Failure to get to sleep is the main symptom which is, as traditional Chinese medicine holds, caused by over—anxiety, impairment of heart and spleen, loss of essence and blood, improper diet and impairment of the stomach and intestines.

Symptoms:

The main symptom of insomnia are failure to fall into sleep or falling asleep with difficulty during the night, or broken sleep and difficulty in getting asleep again. Insomnia of the type "timidity due to insufficiency of Qi and deficiency of blood of the heart" has the additional symptoms of palpitation, dreaminess, liability to wake, vexation, liability to be frightened, night sweating, red margin of the tongue, and taut and fine pulse. Insomnia of the type "deficiency of Qi and blood in the heart and spleen" has the following additional symptoms: palpitation, amnesia, fatigue, poor appetite, pale and dry face, thin and whitish tongue fur, and fine and weak pulse. Insomnia of the type "breakdown of the normal physiological coordination between the heart and the kidney" has the additional symptoms of dizziness, amnesia, tinnitus, palpitation, soreness in loins and knees, oneirogmus, reddened tongue with less coating, and fine and rapid pulse. Insomnia of the type "incoordination between the spleen and the stomach" has the following additional symptoms:

fullness and distention in the stomach and abdomen, belching, difficulty in falling asleep, difficulty in moving bowels, yellowish and greasy tongue fur, and heavy, slippery and rapid pulse.

Treatment:

1. Self Treatment with *Qigong* Exercise

(1) Practise Psychosomatic Relaxation Exercise and Head—Face Exercise as well.

(2) Patients with insomnia of the "timidity due to insufficiency of *Qi* and deficiency of blood of the heart" type, in addition, may practise Heart Regulation Exercise; patients with insomnia of the "deficiency of *Qi* and blood in the heart and spleen" type may practise Heart Regulation Exercise and Spleen Regulation Exercise; patients with insomnia of the "breakdown of the normal physiological coordination between the heart and the kidney" type may practise the Exercise for Ascending and Descending *Yin* and *Yang*, or practise Heart Regulation Exercise and Kidney Regulation Exercise; patients with insomnia of the "incoordination between the spleen and the stomach" type may practise Spleen Regulation Exercise and Automatic *Qi* Circulation Exercise.

2. Treatment with Out—going *Qi*

(1) Tap, press and knead digitally *Dazhui* (Du 14), *Baihui* (Du 20) and *Taiyang* (Extra 2); push and knead *Hanyan* (G.B.4) and *Shuaigu* (G.B. 8); tap and knead *Ganshu* (U.B. 18), *Shenshu* (U.B. 23), *Guanyuan* (Ren 4) and *Qihai* (Ren 6). These procedures may help open through the points and dredge the channels.

(2) Emit *Qi*, with flat—palm gesture and vibrating manipulation, towards the points of *Baihui* (Du 20) and *Dazhui*

(Du 14) respectively for a period of 8 or 16 normal respiration; emit Qi towards *Zhongwan* (Ren 12) and *Guanyuan* (Ren 14) respectively for a period of 8 – 16 normal respiration. Then, emit Qi (with hands off the point) towards *Baihui* (Du 20) with flat-palm gesture and pushing-leading manipulation, and guide Qi to flow to the two points of *Yongquan* (K. 1) along the Kidney Channel. The patient should concentrate his mind on *Yongquan* (K. 1) too.

(3) Again, tap digitally and knead *Baihui* (Du 20) and *Taiyang* (Extra 2), push *Hanyan* (G.B. 4) and *Shuaigu* (G.B. 8), and tap digitally *Baihui* (Du 20) and *Dazhui* (Du 14). Sway the upper extremities.

(4) To treat patients with insomnia of the type "timidity due to insufficiency of Qi and deficiency of blood of the heart", emit Qi, in addition, with middle-finger-propping gesture and vibrating manipulation, towards each of the points of *Xinshu* (U.B. 15), *Ganshu* (U.B. 18) and *Juque* (Ren 14) for a period of 14 normal respiration, and guide Qi, with flat-palm gesture and pushing-leading manipulation, to flow along the Heart Channel and the Gall-Bladder Channel to get the functional activities of Qi balanced. To treat patients with insomnia of the type "breakdown of the normal physiological coordination between the heart and the kidney", emit Qi, in addition, with middle-finger-propping gesture and vibrating manipulation, towards *Shenshu* (U.B. 23) and *Xinshu* (U.B. 15) for a period of 14 normal respiration respectively, and then, with flat-palm gesture and pushing-leading manipulation, guide Qi to flow along the Heart Channel and Kidney Channel to normalize the functional activities of Qi. To treat patients

with insomnia of the type "deficiency of *Qi* and blood in the heart and spleen", emit *Qi,* in addition, with middle–finger–propping gesture and vibrating manipulation, towards *Pishu* (U.B. 20) and *Xinshu* (U.B. 15) respectively for a period of 14 normal respiration, and guide *Qi,* with flat–palm gesture and pushing–leading manipulation,to flow along the Spleen Channel to get the functional activities of *Qi* normalized. To treat patients with insomnia of the type "incoordination between the spleen and the stomach", emit *Qi,* with middle–finger–propping gesture and vibrating manipulation, towards *Pishu* (U.B.20) and *Weishu* (U.B.21) respectively for a period of 14 normal respiration, and then with flat–palm gesture and pushing–leading manipulation, guide *Qi* to flow along the Stomach Channel to get the functional activities of *Qi* normalized.

5.25 Hypertension

Hypertension means a state in which blood pressure is often higher than 18.7 / 12 KPa (140 / 90 mmHg) at rest. Traditional Chinese medicine believes that hypertension is caused by incoordination of the liver and kidney, excess of *Yin* and *Yang,*or up–invasion of phlegm–dampness.

Symptoms:

Patients with hypertension of the type "flaming–up of the liver–fire" have the symptoms of headache, fullness of head, flushed face and eyes, dry mouth, vexation, liability to anger, constipation, yellowish tongue fur, and taut, rapid and forceful pulse. Patients with hypertension of "deficiency of the liver–*Yin* and kidney–*Yin*" type may have the following symptoms: vertigo, tinnitus, lassitude in loins and legs, palpitation, insomnia, deep reddened tongue, and taut, thin and rapid pulse. In addition, symptoms of phlegm-dampness, e.g., oppressed feeling in the chest, numbness of the exetremities, obesity in appearance, and taut, slippery pulse may sometimes be seen in patients with hypertension of the above-mentioned two types.

Treatment:

1. Self Treatment with *Qigong* Exercise

(1) Practise Psychosomatic Relaxation Exercise as well as Head-Face Exercise, Neck Exercise, Upper-Limb Exercise and Exercise of the Lower Limbs.

(2) Patients with hypertension of "flaming-up of the liver-fire" type should, in addition, practise "rubbing the hypochondrium and '*Xu*' *Qi*" included in the Liver Regulation Exercise. Patients with hypertension of "deficiency of liver- *Yin* and kidney-*Yin*" type should, in addition, practise Kidney Regulation Exercise and Liver Regulation Exercise.

2. Treatment with Out-going *Qi*

(1) Press and knead *Lanmen* (the ileocecal junction), *Zhongwan* (Ren 12) and *Guanyuan* (Ren 4); push *Tianmen* (life pass), *Kangong* and *Taiyang* (Extra 2); tap and knead digitally *Pishu* (U.B. 20), *Weishu* (U.B.21), *Ganshu* (U.B. 18), *Danshu* (U.B. 19) and *Zusanli* (St.36); knead the Urinary Bladder Channel of both sides.

(2) Emit *Qi*, with flat-palm gesture and vibrating manipulation, towards *Baihui* (Du 20), *Dazhui* (Du 14), *Mingmen* (Du 4), *Zhongwan* (Ren 12) and *Guanyuan* (Ren 4) for a period of 8 or 16 normal respiration respectively; emit *Qi*,

with vibrating manipulation, towards *Zhongwan* (Ren 12) for a period of 8 normal respiration; emit *Qi*, with flat-palm gesture and pushing-pulling-quivering- leading manipulation (hand off the treated parts), towards *Baihui* (Du 20) and *Dantian*. Then, guide *Qi*, with pushing-pulling-leading manipulation, to flow to the lower limbs along the Stomach Channel to render the functional activities of *Qi* excessive in the upper and deficient in the lower; guide *Qi*, with the same manipulation, to flow to the extremity ends along the Large Intestine Channel of Hand-*Yangming* till the functional activities of *Qi* get normalized.

(3) To treat patients with hypertension of "flaming-up of the liver-fire" type, flat-palm gesture and pushing-pulling-rotating manipulation should be applied to emit *Qi* towards *Ganshu* (U.B. 18), *Shenshu* (U.B. 23) and *Dantian* and, with a rotating manipulation, guide *Qi* to flow accordingly. This may help *Yin* and supress hyperactive *Yang*. To treat patients with hypertension of the "deficiency of liver-*Yin* and kidney-*Yin*" type, flat-palm gesture and vibrating manipulation should be used to emit *Qi* towards *Shenshu* (U.B. 23) and *Dantian* to help nourish the liver-*Yin* and kidney-*Yin*.

5.26 Cervical Spondylopathy

Also called retrograde cervical spondylosis, it is common in people over the age of 40. Cervical spondylopathy is, as traditional Chinese medicine holds, caused by wind-cold-dampness, trauma, over-exertion, and failure of blood to nourish the muscles which is caused by the insufficiency of *Qi* and blood due to old age.

Symptoms:

Clinically, symptoms of cervical spondylopathy are miscellaneous; however, those such as pain or numbing pain in the neck, shoulders (including the surrounding), upper part of the back and chest and upper extremities due to irritation or compression of cervical nerve roots are common. Cervical overstrain or exopathic cold may serve as factors inducing this disease or worsening its symptoms. If the spinal cord is irritated or compressed, symptoms of numbness and weakness of the lower extremities, and staggering gait may appear; while if vertebral artery is irritated or compressed, vertigo and dizziness may appear.

Treatment:

1. Self Treatment with *Qigong* Exercise

(1) Practise Neck Exercise, Shoulder—Arm Exercise and Brocade Exercise in Six Forms.

(2) Patients with vertigo and dizziness may, in addition, practise Psychosomatic Relaxation Exercise, Head—Face Exercise and Liver Regulation Exercise; patients with weakness of the lower limbs and staggering gait should, additionally, practise Exercise of the Lower Limbs and Exercise for Ascending and Descending *Yin* and *Yang*.

2. Treatment with Out—going *Qi*

(1) Press and knead *Fengchi* (G.B. 20), *Fengfu* (Du 16), *Tianzhu* (U.B. 10), *Jianzhongshu* (S.I. 15), *Jianwaishu* (S.I. 14), *Jiquan* (H. 1), *Quchi* (L.I. 11), *Hegu* (L.I. 4), *Shaohai* (H. 3) and *Xiaohai* (S.I. 8) to promote the flow of *Qi* and blood.

(2) Emit *Qi*, with flat—palm gesture and vibrating manipulation, towards *Dazhui* (Du 14) for a period of 16 normal respi-

ration, and with flat-palm gesture and pushing-pulling-leading manipulation, towards *Dazhui* (Du 14) as well as the neck.Then guide *Qi* to flow to the fingertips along the Three-*Yang* Channels of Hand.

(3) Again press and knead the points mentioned above. Conduct patting, taping, rocking and foulage manipulations to end the treatment.

5.27 Hemiplegia

Hemiplegia is the sequela of apoplexy caused by exopathic wind or upstirring of liver.

Symptoms:

Wry mouth with distorted eyes, hemiparalysis, stiff tongue and flaccidity of the hand and foot are the marked symptoms.

Treatment:

1. Self Treatment with *Qigong* Exercise

(1) Try to promote movements of the affected limbs.

(2) Gently pat the affected limb with the fist of the healthy side, 3 − 5 times from the upper to the lower part.

(3) Hold and move the affected limb with the hand of the healthy limb, moving upward and inward when inhaling and moving to its original place when exhaling. Imagine that *Qi* is flowing to the affected limb at the same time.

(4) Practise Upper-Limb Exercise, Exercise of the Lower Limbs and Head-Face Exercise.

2. Treatment with Out-going *Qi*

(1) Press and knead *Hegu* (L.I.4), *Jiache* (St.6), *Neiguan* (P.6), *Quchi*(L.I.11), *Yanglingquan* (G.B. 34) and *Weizhong* (U.B.

40); pinch the fingertips and the sides of the nails of the affected limb.

(2) Press and knead the Urinary Bladder Channel from the upper to the lower part for 6 − 7 times.

(3) Emit *Qi*, with flat−palm or sword−thrust hand gesture and pushing−pulling− leading manipulation, towards *Yintang* (Extra 1) and *Baihui* (du 20), then guide *Qi* to flow downward.

(4) Emit *Qi*, with flat−palm gesture and pushing−pulling−leading manipulation, towards *Dazhui* (Du 14), *Fengmen* (U.B.12), *Ganshu* (U.B. 18) and *Shenshu* (U.B. 23), then guide *Qi* to flow via the neck from the left part of the head to the right part of the body and vice versa. This may help normalize the functional activities of *Qi*.

5.28 Myopia

Myopia is common in youngsters. It is believed that this disease is related to improper lightening, improper posture and successive long−time reading.

Symptoms:

To victims of myopia, all objects in distance are blurred although nearby objects are clear.

Treatment:

1. Self Treatment with *Qigong* Exercise

Practise Exercise for Soothing the Liver to Improve the Acuity of Vision, as well as Eye Exercise.

2. Treatment with Out−going *Qi*

(1) Press and knead *Jingming* (U.B. 1), *Qiuhou* (Extra 4), *Yintang* (Extra 1), *Taiyang* (Extra 2), *Fengchi* (G.B.

20) , *Hegu* (L.I. 4) and *Guangming* (G.B. 37) .
(2) Single—finger—miditation or sword—thrust and pushing—pulling manipulation, or middle—finger—propping gesture and vibrating manipulation are used to emit *Qi* towards the points of *Jingming* (U.B. 1) , *Ganshu* (U.B. 18) and *Shenshu* (U.B. 23) respectively for a period of 14 normal respiration.
(3) Emit *Qi,* with flat—palm gesture and pushing—pulling—leading manipulation, towards the eyes, then guide *Qi* to flow along the Gallbladder Channel, to make the functional activities of *Qi* normalized.

5.29 Infantile Convulsion

Infantile convulsion is usually caused by fright.
Symptoms:
Disphoria, listlessness, night crying, poor appetite, diarrhoea and fever are the symptoms of infantile convulsion.
Treatment:
1. Knead *Xiaotianxin* (a massage point, at the root of the palm and the depression between the thenar eminence major and thenar eminence minor) and nip the Heart Channel, the Liver Channel, the joints of the five fingers of each hand and the points *Yintang* (Extra 1) and *Baihui* (Du 20) .
2. Use flat—palm gesture and pushing—pulling—leading manipulation to emit *Qi* towards the fontanel and *Baihui* (Du 20) and then, to guide *Qi* to flow to *Dantian* along the *Ren* Channel to "get *Qi* back to its origin" as it is called.
3. Use flat—palm gesture and pushing—pulling—leading manipulation to emit *Qi* towards *Dazhui* (Du 14) , *Xinshu* (U.B.

15) and *Ganshu* (U.B. 18) and then, to get *Qi* normalized in the Urinary Bladder CHannel and the *Du* Channel.

5.30 Infantile Diarrhoea

Infantile diarrhoea is usually caused by pathogenic cold–dampness and summer–heat, or by improper diet and weakness of the spleen and the stomach.

Symptoms:

Loose stool, frequent defecation and indigestion are the general symptoms of infantile diarrhoea of all types. The symptoms of infantile diarrhoea vary with the type of the disease. Patients of cold–dampness type have the symptoms of watery stool with abundant foams, borborygmus and abdominal pain; patients of damp–heat type have the symptoms of defecating upon abdominal pain, spouting diarrhoea, yellow, hot and foul stool, fever and thirst; patients of improper– diet type have the symptoms of abdominal fullness and pain, pain which may be relieved after defecating and foul stool; patients of spleen–deficiency type have the symptoms of protracted diarrhoea, frequent attacks and defecating after meals.

Treatment:

1. Press and knead *Pishu* (U.B. 20), *Weishu* (U.B. 21), *Dachangshu* (U.B. 25), *Tianshu* (St. 25), *Zhongwan* (Ren 12) and *Dantian*.

2. Flat–palm gesture and vibrating manipulation are used to emit *Qi* towards each of the points of *Zhongwan* (Ren 12), *Tianshu* (St. 25) and *Guanyuan* (Ren 4) for a period of 8 or 16 normal respiration, then use flat–palm gesture and

pushing-pulling-rotating manipulation to emit *Qi* towards the whole abdomen and to guide *Qi* to whirl in different directions decided by whether tonification or purgation is required.

3. To treat patients with symptoms of "heat of excess type", flat-palm gesture and pulling-leading manipulation are used to emit *Qi* towards *Zhongwan* (Ren 12) and to guide the pathogenic factors out of the body.

4. To treat patients with symptoms of "weakness of the spleen and stomach" type, flat-palm gesture and pushing-locating manipulation are used to emit *Qi* towards *Zhongwan* (Ren 12) and *Dantian* to tonify primordial *Qi*.

(Sun Xigang)

8

医学气功

序

　　《英汉实用中医药大全》即将问世,吾为之高兴。

　　歧黄之道,历经沧桑,永盛不衰。吾中华民族之强盛,由之。世界医学之丰富和发展,亦由之。然而,世界民族之差异,国别之不同,语言之障碍,使中医中药的传播和交流受到了严重束缚。当前,世界各国人民学习、研究、运用中医药的热潮方兴未艾。为使吾中华民族优秀文化遗产之一的歧黄之道走向世界,光大其业,为世界人民造福,徐象才君集省内外精英于一堂,主持编译了《英汉实用中医药大全》。是书之问世将使海内外同道欢呼雀跃。

　　世界医学发展之日,当是歧黄之道光大之时。

　　吾欣然序之。

中华人民共和国卫生部副部长
兼国家中医药管理局局长
世界针灸学会联合会主席
中国科学技术协会委员
中华全国中医学会副会长
中国针灸学会会长　　　　胡　熙　明

一九八九年十二月

序

　　中华民族有同疾病长期作斗争的光辉历程，故而有自己的传统医学——中国医药学。中国医药学有一套完整的从理论到实践的独特科学体系。几千年来，它不但被完好地保存下来，而且得到了发扬光大。它具有疗效显著、副作用小等优点，是人们防病治病，强身健体的有效工具。

　　任何一个国家在医学进步中所取得的成就，都是人类共同的财富，是没有国界的。医学成果的交流比任何其他科学成果的交流都应进行得更及时，更准确。我从事中医工作30多年来，一直盼望着有朝一日中国医药学能全面走向世界，为全人类解除病痛疾苦做出其应有的贡献。但由于用外语表达中医难度较大，中国医药学对外传播的速度一直不能令人满意。

　　山东中医学院的徐象才老师发起并主持了大型系列丛书《英汉实用中医药大全》的编译工作。这个工作是一项巨大工程，是一种大型科研活动，是一个大胆的尝试，是一件新事物。对徐象才老师及与其合作的全体编译者夜以继日地长期工作所付出的艰苦劳动，克服重重困难所表现出的坚韧不拔的毅力，以及因此而取得的重大成绩，我甚为敬佩。作为一个中医界的领导者，对他们的工作给予全力支持是我应尽的责任。

　　我相信《英汉实用中医药大全》无疑会在中国医学史和世界科学技术史上找到它应有的位置。

中华全国中医学会常务理事
山东省卫生厅副厅长
张奇文
1990年3月

出 版 前 言

　　中国医药学是我中华民族优秀文化遗产之一，建国以来由于党和国家对中医药采取了正确的政策，使中医药理论宝库不断得到了发掘整理，取得了巨大的成绩。当前，世界各国人民对中国医药学的学习和研究热潮日益高涨。为促进这一热潮更加蓬勃的发展，为使中国医药学能更好地为全人类解除病痛服务，就必须促进中医中药在世界范围内的传播和交流，而要使这一传播和交流进行得更及时、更准确，就必须首先排除语言障碍。因此，编写一套英汉对照的中医药基本知识的书籍，供国内外学习、研究中医药时使用，已成为国内外医药学界和医药学教育界许多人士的迫切需要。

　　多年来，在卫生部门的号召下，在"中医英语表达研究"方面，已经作出了一些可喜的成绩。《英汉实用中医药大全》的编辑出版就是在调查上述研究工作的历史和现状的基础上，继续对中医药英语表达作较系统、较全面的研究，以适应中国医药学对外传播交流的需要。

　　这套"大全"的版本为英汉对照，共有21个分册，一个分册介绍论述中国医药学的一个分科。在编著上注意了中医药汉文稿的编写特色，在内容上注意了科学性、实用性、全面性和简明易读。汉文稿的执笔撰写者主要是有20年以上实践经验的副教授、教授、副主任医师和主任医师。各分册汉文稿撰写完成后，均经各学科专家逐一审订。各分册英文主译、主审主要是国内既懂中医又懂英语的权威人士，中医院校的英语教师和医药卫生部门的专业翻译人员。英译稿脱稿后，经过了复审、终审，有些译稿还召开全国22所院校和单位人员参加的英译稿统稿定稿研讨会,对英译稿进行细致的研讨和推敲,对如何较全面、较系统、较准确地用英语表达中国医药学进行了探讨,从而推动整个译文达到较高水平,因此,这套"大全"可供中医院校高年级学生作为原读教材使用。

这套"大全"的编纂得到了国家教育委员会、国家中医药管理局、山东省教育委员会、山东省卫生厅等各部门有关领导的支持。在国家教委高等教育司的指导下,成立了《英汉实用中医药大全》编译领导委员会。还得到了全国许多中医院校和中药生产厂家领导的支持。

希望这套"大全"的出版,对中医院校加强中医英语教学,对国内卫生界培养外向型中医药人才,以及在推动世界各国人民对中医药学习和研究方面,都能产生良好的影响。

高等教育出版社
1990年3月

前 言

《英汉实用中医药大全》是一部以中医基本理论为基础,以中医临床为重点,较为全面系统、简明扼要、易读实用的中级英汉学术性著作。它的主要读者是:中医药院校高年级学生和中青年教师,中医院的中青年医生和中医药科研单位的科研人员,从事中医对外函授工作的人员和出国讲学或行医的中医人员,西学中人员,来华学习中医的外国留学生和各类进修人员。

由于中国医药学为我中华民族之独有,因此,英译便成了本"大全"编译工作的重点。为确保译文能准确表达中医的确切含义,我们邀集熟悉中医的英语人员、医学专业翻译人员、懂英语的中医药人员乃至医古文人员于一堂,共同翻译、共同对译文进行研讨推敲的集体翻译法,最后,又请在华学习中医或从事英语教学的母语是英语的外籍人士对译稿进行了文字润色。这样,就把众人之长融进了译文质量之中。然而,即使这样,也难确保译文都能尽如人意。汉文稿虽反映了中国医药学的精髓和概貌,但也难能十全十美。我衷心地盼望读者能提出批评和建议,以便再版时修改。

参加本"大全"编、译、审工作的人员达200余名,他们来自全国28个单位,其中有山东、北京、上海、天津、南京、浙江、安徽、河南、湖北、广西、贵阳、甘肃、成都、山西、长春等15所中医学院,还有中国中医研究院,山东省中医药研究所等中医药科研单位。

山东省教育委员会把本"大全"的编译列入了科研计划并拨发了科研经费,山东省卫生厅和一些中药生产厂家也给了很大支持,济南中药厂的资助为编译工作提供了条件。

本"大全"的编译成功是全体编、译、审者集体劳动的结晶，是各有关单位主管领导支持的结果。在"大全"出版之际，我诚挚地感谢全体编译审者的真诚合作，感谢许多专家、教授、各级领导的热情支持。

愿本"大全"的出版能在培养通晓英语的中医人才和使中医早日全面走向世界方面起到所设想的作用。

主编　徐象才

于山东中医学院

一九九〇年三月

目 录

说明 ·· 261
1 概论 ·· 263
  1.1 气功的概念与特点 ······················ 263
  1.2 气功的发展概要 ·························· 264
  1.3 练功的基本原则 ·························· 267
    1.3.1 动静结合 ······························ 267
    1.3.2 松静自然 ······························ 267
    1.3.3 意气相随 ······························ 268
    1.3.4 练养相兼 ······························ 268
    1.3.5 循序渐进 ······························ 268
2 气功三调 ·· 270
  2.1 调身 ·· 270
    2.1.1 坐式 ··································· 270
    2.1.2 卧式 ··································· 271
    2.1.3 站式 ··································· 272
    2.1.4 锻炼姿势的要领 ······················ 273
  2.2 调息 ·· 274
    2.2.1 自然呼吸 ······························ 275
    2.2.2 顺腹式呼吸 ··························· 275
    2.2.3 逆腹式呼吸 ··························· 275
    2.2.4 其它呼吸法 ··························· 275
    2.2.5 锻炼呼吸的要领 ······················ 276
  2.3 调心 ·· 276
  2.4 常用穴窍 ····································· 277

2.5	练功中应注意的问题	279
3	**功法**	**281**
3.1	放松功	281
3.2	内养功	282
3.3	强壮功	283
3.4	头面功	284
3.5	眼功	287
3.6	鼻齿功	288
3.7	耳功	290
3.8	颈项功	291
3.9	肩臂功	293
3.10	胸胁功	294
3.11	腹部功	295
3.12	腰部功	296
3.13	下肢功	297
3.14	理心功	298
3.15	理脾功	302
3.16	理肺功	304
3.17	理肝功	306
3.18	理肾功	309
3.19	周天自转功	311
3.20	周天功	312
3.21	疏肝明目功	313
3.22	养肾回春功	317
3.23	采日精月华功	319
3.24	倒阳功	320
3.25	回精还液功	322
3.26	涤秽功	323
3.27	铁裆功	324

3.28	升降阴阳导引功	330
3.29	通任督导引功	331
3.30	六段锦	333
3.31	延年九转功	338
3.32	易筋经	339

4 发放外气 350
4.1 练气 350
4.1.1 静功练气 350
4.1.2 动功练气 352

4.2 导气 361
4.2.1 合掌震桩导气 361
4.2.2 一指禅导气 361
4.2.3 对掌推拉导气 362
4.2.4 三点拉线导气 362
4.2.5 三点求圆导气 363
4.2.6 腾跃爆发导气 364
4.2.7 点射形导气 364
4.2.8 螺旋形导气 365
4.2.9 冷热导气 365

4.3 发气 366
4.3.1 发气手式 366
4.3.2 发气手法 368
4.3.3 发气中的气形 370
4.3.4 气感 371
4.3.5 气效应 372
4.3.6 收功 373

5 治疗 374
5.1 气功偏差 374
5.1.1 气血逆乱 375

  5.1.2 气滞血瘀 ………………………………………… 375
  5.1.3 真气走失 ………………………………………… 376
  5.1.4 神昏颠倒 ………………………………………… 377
  5.1.5 练功中暂时反应的处理 ………………………… 378
 5.2 昏厥 ……………………………………………………… 378
 5.3 感冒 ……………………………………………………… 379
 5.4 胃脘痛 …………………………………………………… 380
 5.5 阑尾炎 …………………………………………………… 381
 5.6 胆道疾患 ………………………………………………… 382
 5.7 呃逆 ……………………………………………………… 384
 5.8 胃下垂 …………………………………………………… 384
 5.9 泄泻 ……………………………………………………… 385
 5.10 便秘 …………………………………………………… 386
 5.11 胁痛 …………………………………………………… 387
 5.12 支气管炎 ……………………………………………… 388
 5.13 支气管哮喘 …………………………………………… 389
 5.14 心悸 …………………………………………………… 390
 5.15 遗精 …………………………………………………… 391
 5.16 阳痿 …………………………………………………… 392
 5.17 痛经 …………………………………………………… 393
 5.18 慢性盆腔炎 …………………………………………… 394
 5.19 子宫脱垂 ……………………………………………… 394
 5.20 乳痈 …………………………………………………… 395
 5.21 落枕 …………………………………………………… 396
 5.22 腰腿痛 ………………………………………………… 397
 5.23 头痛 …………………………………………………… 398
 5.24 失眠 …………………………………………………… 399
 5.25 高血压病 ……………………………………………… 400
 5.26 颈椎病 ………………………………………………… 401

5.27 半身不遂 …………………………………… 402
5.28 近视眼 ……………………………………… 403
5.29 小儿惊症 …………………………………… 403
5.30 小儿腹泻 …………………………………… 404

说　明

　　《医学气功》一书是《英汉实用中医药大全》中的第八分册。

　　气功疗法主要有气功自控疗法和气功外气疗法两大部分。前者是患者通过自我练功而达到健身和治病的目的；后者是练气功有素者发放外气为患者治病的一种医疗方法。

　　本分册共有概论、气功三调、功法、发放外气、治疗等五章，简要介绍气功的基础知识，重点讲解了气功自控治病的功法以及外气疗法的练气、导气和发气等。

　　治疗是气功的临床应用。书中除简要介绍疾病的病因病理和症状外，详细讲解了气功辩证施治的功法和发气方法，由此可见，这本书既可供国内外医务工作者，气功爱好者学习参考，也是患者练气功自控治病的良师益友。

　　本分册汉文稿的编写得到了山东中医学院医古文教研室主任邵冠勇教授的热情帮助。

编　者

1 概　　论

1.1　气功的概念与特点

　　气功是中华民族优秀文化遗产之一，它是人们通过意念、呼吸、姿势的锻炼，调节机体的生理状况，达到防治疾病、养生健身、益寿延年目的。练气功有素者将内气发放于外，为患者治疗疾病，叫外气疗法，也属气功的范畴。

　　气功是练气的功夫。气，是指"真气"，也叫"内气"。中医学认为，真气是人体生命活动的动力，因此气功所指的练气，就是锻炼真气。导引是气功中的一种特殊锻炼方法，中医学又称为导引按摩，它是针对健身或防治某种疾病而设计的一种练功方法。一般是通过一定姿势、呼吸、意念，还要结合某些按摩手法来进行综合锻炼。另外，当练气达到一定程度，自感体内有气在流动时，再通过一定意念的导引，使气向一定的方向流动也称之为导引。如内养功、强壮功、养气功、周天功是以练内气（真气）为主的功法；而铁裆功、部位导引功、理五脏等功法则多是配合一定的按摩手法，这是用来治疗某种疾病的功法。

　　气功的特点之一，是辨证施功。在选择功法时，既注意改善人的整个机体功能，又强调针对疾病的具体情况。如练静功，主要是通过姿势、精神、内脏的放松，呼吸的调整，排除杂念，意守丹田，或意守某一部位，从而达到练气和积气，增强体质，延年益寿的目的。而有某些疾病的人，则要选择针对性强的功法进行锻炼。如心气虚弱而出现心慌、气短等症状者，则可选择铁裆功来锻炼方能较快的收到疗效。根据个人的体质以及疾病的寒热虚实等情况来练功，中医叫辨证施治。

气功的另一特点是强调自我锻炼。古人说："流水不腐，户枢不蠹"。《内经》中指出的"导引按跷"主要是通过自身主动的运动肢体，按摩导引气脉而达到健身治病目的的一种方法。这种方法在很大程度上优于被动的按摩、针灸、服药等疗法，因为它是强调调动自身的正气和潜能来防治疾病的。

气功还有简单，易行，照书，看图可以锻炼，收效快，疗效好等特点。

1.2 气功的发展概要

气功作为医疗保健方法，已有很长的历史。相传早在4000多年前的唐尧时代，人们就已经知道用"舞"的方法治病了。《吕氏春秋·古乐》中说："昔陶唐氏之始，阴多滞伏而湛积，水道壅塞，不行其原，民气郁阏而滞着，筋骨瑟缩不达，故作为舞以宣导之。"古人在与大自然斗争的长期实践中，逐渐体会到：一定的动作，呼吸和发音的声调，可以调节人体的某些机能，诸如学习飞禽走兽的攀缘、顾盼、跳跃、展翅动作能宣导气机，"嘿"声能降力发力，"哈"声能散热，"嘘"声可以止痛等等，古老的气功就以此产生了。

春秋战国时期，诸子蜂起，百家争鸣。人们总结了前人的经验，把人们对自然、社会以及人自身生命的认识推进到理论的新高度，气功也在这个背景上系统化，形成了独立的理论体系。例如：《管子》中说："精者，气之精也"；"心之在体，君之位也"；"气者，体之充也"。《孟子》中提出"存其心，养其性"，《荀子》中指出"虚一而静"。诸子百家各自提出了相应的养生主张，明确提出了人身三宝，精气神的概念。《庄子》有"吹呴呼吸，吐故纳新，熊经鸟伸"的肢体活动与呼吸配合的气功健身治疗方法。

秦汉时期医疗技术有了很大的发展。在中医经典著作《内经》中就把"导引"、"行气"、"按跷"等方法作为重要的治疗措施，并且指出"恬惔虚无，独立守神，肌肉若一"。《素问·遗篇刺法论》中还具体的记载了一则导引治病的方法："肾有久病者，可以寅时面向南，净神不乱思，闭气不息七遍，以引颈咽气顺之，如咽甚硬物，如此七遍后，饵舌下津令无数。"

1973年以湖南长沙马王堆三号汉墓出土的文物中，发现了西汉时期的帛书《却谷食气篇》和帛画《导引图》。前者的内容是"导引行气"法，后者是44幅彩绘"导引图"，图中绘有人模仿狼、猴、猿、熊、鹤、鹞、鹞运动的图象。这说明我国在西汉初期，就已经用彩色图谱的形式来传授气功了。

东汉末年的两位大医学家张仲景，华佗都曾提到气功。张仲景在《金匮要略》中说："四肢才觉重滞，即导引吐纳、针灸膏摩，勿令九窍闭塞。"华佗创作了著名的医疗保健气功"五禽戏"一直流传至现在。

魏晋南北朝时期不但在气功养生方面有了很大的发展，而且将气功外气应用疗病。晋人张湛所著《养生要集》列养生大要十项，其中"啬神"、"爱气"、"养形"、"导引"都是气功的内容。晋代医学家葛洪在他的《抱扑子》一书中，记录了各种长生的方术。南北朝时的医学家陶弘景编写了《养性延命录》，辑录了不少古代气功的方法与理论，在其"服气疗病"和"导引按摩"两部分中详细的介绍了一些动功和静功的内容。《晋书》记载幸灵用外气治愈吕猗母十余年的"痿痹病"取得了"遂能行"的效果而闻名于世，于是有"百姓奔趣，水陆辐辏，从之如云"的记载。

隋唐时期气功被广泛应用于临床医疗。在《诸病源候论》、《备急千金要方》、《外台秘要》中均收集了丰富的气功治疗方法，而且多是一病一法，辨证施功。其中《诸病源候论》一书就收载气功疗病260余条。在《备急千金要方》中还保存了完整的"天竺国按摩婆罗门法"与"老子按摩法"等气功导引按摩保健功法。唐《幻真先生服内之气诀》中记载了"布气诀"。介绍了发放外气的要领、放法等。晚唐无名氏所著《无能子》也有无能子布气治愈其心友禺中子的心痛病的记载。

宋金元时期，道教内丹术兴起，古代气功开始融合其中的某些部分，促进了医疗气功的发展。如《圣济总录》中列导引、服气两部分，记载了不少古代气功资料，在金元四大医家的著作里，也有很多气功的记载。如李东垣在《兰室秘藏》中说："当病之时，宜安心静坐，以养其气"。刘河间在《素问玄机病源式》中提到用六字诀治病，朱丹溪在《丹溪心法》中提到"气滞痿厥寒热者，治以导引"，张子和在他的《儒门事亲》中指出，导引是汗法之一等等。

进入明清时期，气功发展的特点是更广泛地为医家所掌握、所应用，所以在医学著作中这方面的资料也就更多了。在王履所著的《医经溯回集》，万全著的《万密斋医书十种》，徐春甫编的《古今医统大全》等著作中都有很丰富的气功资料。伟大的医学家李时珍对古代气功更有深刻认识。他在《奇经八脉考》中明确的指出："内景隧道，唯返观者能照察之。"这一著名论断说明了练功与经络的关系。

中华人民共和国成立以后，气功得到重视和发展。1955年在唐山建立了气功疗养院；刘贵珍和胡耀贞继承前人练功经验结合自己的体会，写出《气功疗法实践》与《气功及保健功》，介绍了内养功、保健功等功法，对全国气功研究的发展作出了贡献。

自1978年以来，全国各地医务工作者和气功师在广大人民群众中积极推广、普及气功健身防病，取得了很好的效果。一些科技工作者不仅从现代医学角度对气功进行生理、生化方面的研究，而且还从多科学入手进行"外气"物理效应的研究，探讨人体"气"的本质，从此，气功的研究和应用进入了一个新的历史时期。各省市相继成立了气功研究会，很多省市医疗单位建立气功医院、气功科，从事气功研究、教学和医疗工作。习练气功、研究气功蔚然成风。在普及与研究的同时,广大气功工作者及时总结经验,仅仅十多年的时间,就有《气功杂志》、《气功与科学》、《中华气功》、《中国气功》、《东方气功》等气功专业杂志出版,还出版了《气功疗法集锦》、《新气功疗法》、《中国气功学》、《气功养生学概要》等气功书籍。

1.3 练功的基本原则

1.3.1 动静结合

从姿势的动静来说,练功中肢体运动者称动功,肢体不动者称静功。练功要选择适合于自己身体情况的功法来锻炼,练静功目的是练气积气,使丹田气机充实,进一步锻练可以开通小周天。练动功则能疏通气机,使四肢百骸经络通畅,使真气直达病所,有助于疾病的治疗。

在练动功或静功时,要掌握"动中静"、"静中动"的原则。练动功时,在保持外形手法动的条件下,思想集中,注意着动作,以及气行经络的效应。在练静功时,愈是安静和放松时,气行经络的效应就愈能体会到,要正确体会这种动的感觉,就能有助于思想集中,排除杂念,提高练功的质量。

1.3.2 松静自然

松是指练功活动中要放松,不但要肢体放松,还要做到精神放松,因为只有精神不紧张,才能使肢体放松,但是这里所指的松,不是松懈或松散,而是在觉醒状态下,在意念的支配下做到松而不懈,松中有紧,紧而不僵。

静是指练功过程中,保持情绪安宁。静只是相对的,绝对的静是不存在的。气功的入静与自然睡眠和普通休息不同,它是在觉醒状态下的一种特殊的安静状态,也可以说,它是在安静状态下的一种特殊的觉醒。

1.3.3　意气相随

意气相随，是指练功中意气不离。在练功时不能偏面的强调以意引气，硬要使呼吸拉的"柔、细、匀、长"，而不是经过锻练自然形成的一种"柔细匀长"的呼吸，或不适当的要求腹式呼吸，故意鼓肚挺胸，失去自然。或者体内出现了气动的现象，硬是以意念领其向某方向运行，而不是顺乎自然，在锻练中自然形成。清代薛阳桂在《梅华问答篇》中说："心静自然息调，息调自然神凝，所谓心息相依，息调心定者也"。也不要片面的追求练功的气感，在练功中出现冷、热、麻、胀、痒、轻、重、浮、沉或暖流在一定路线上流动，都不要去追求，或夸张，或硬要想练出这种效果来，这都是不恰当的。

导引功，当手法按摩导引时，一定要手到意到，意到手到，体会手下的感觉，呼吸也要配合好。若感觉不明显，也不要追求，只是将注意力集中在手下即可。

1.3.4　练养相兼

"练"是指在练功时，有意识地摆好姿势，调整身体，内外放松，调整呼吸，排除杂念，运用手法或推或摩等一系列的练功过程。所谓"练"就是在强有力的意识支配下运用呼吸和意念练功。"养"是在练后所出现的静松舒适的入静状态。此时意念呼吸都不要过重，要淡淡的，形成一种静养的状态。

练功中，练与养往往是交替进行，互相促进的。如练完导引功，再练一会养的静功；练静功后再练一会导引功等使其练中有养，或养中有练，练养结合，提高练功的质量。

1.3.5　循序渐进

练气功必须循序渐进，否则欲速则不达，练气功或导引功，首先要选好功法。经过艰苦锻炼，逐渐做到能使内气在自己的意志控制下随姿势、手法、呼吸和意念的活动而进行。

在练功前要先学一些基础知识，要练得很好，不是短时间能做得到的。一般人容易发生这样的偏差：一是急于求成，想一下子就把病治好，练得过多过猛，而造成疲劳，某些部位疼痛、酸胀，或疾病加重，便认为是功法不好，或出了气功偏差问题，而害怕起来，二是松懈散慢，放任自流，朝三暮四，"三天打鱼两天晒网"，久久不出现功夫，不见成效。

所以，在练功中，要根据功法要求，认真的去做，克服客观上的困难，多多体会，坚持不懈的锻炼，就会达到预期的目的。

2 气功三调

2.1 调身

调身又叫姿势、身法等,初练静功或导引功的人掌握好正确的姿势是很重要的。

练功的姿势,从总的方面来说大体可有坐、卧、站、走四类。静功锻炼常用坐、卧、站来进行。导引功常用站、坐、卧、走来进行。本功法常用的姿势有以下几种:

2.1.1 坐式:

(1) 平坐式:端坐在宽平的方凳上,两足平行踏地,距离与

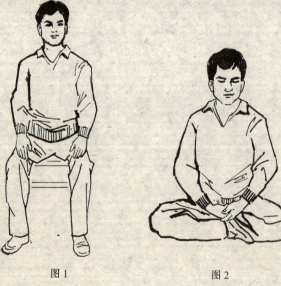

图1　　　　　　　　图2

肩相等。膝关节屈成90度，身体端正，大腿和躯干成90度，手心向下轻轻放在大腿上，两肘自然弯曲，头端正，下颌微收，腰背正直，垂肩含胸，口眼轻闭，舌抵上腭（见图1）。

(2) 盘坐式：两腿交叉盘起，两足放在腿下，稳坐于床上，臀部略垫高一些，身体略向前倾，两手相互轻握，左手在上，右手拇指掐左手子文，左手拇、中指相结合，置于腹前，上半身姿势前倾（见图2）。

2.1.2 卧式

(1) 侧卧式：侧身卧于床上（左右侧卧均可，一般采用左侧卧），上身成微弓形，头略向胸收，平稳着枕，口眼轻闭，舌抵上腭。下侧的手仰掌置于枕上，高低以舒适为宜，上侧手掌腹盖于下侧手掌上，成合掌式，或上侧手指的小指、无名指、中指、食指指尖分别放在下侧小、无名、中、食指的掌指关节横纹上，拇指自然合于下掌虎口外侧。或上侧手臂自然放于身体上侧亦可。下侧小腿自然伸直，上侧的腿自然弯曲，放在下侧腿上（见图3）。

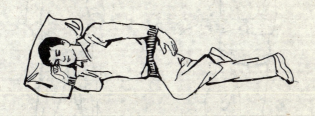

图3

(2) 仰卧式：全身平卧床上，面朝天，头正、四肢自然伸直，两手放于身旁或相叠于腹部，轻闭口眼，舌抵上腭（见图4）。

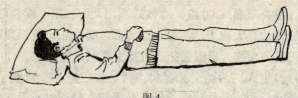

图 4

2.1.3 站式

两脚左右分开,间隔与肩同宽,头端正,腰直,含胸,膝松,两臂抬起微曲。手指自然张开,在胸前或小腹前作抱球状(见图 5);或两手在胸前合掌成佛掌式;或两手下按(见图 6);也可两手放于小腹部相叠(见图 7),或右上肢屈肘于胸前,右手仰掌平膻中穴,左手竖掌,指尖向上,掌心对准左手小鱼际成乾坤掌式(见图 8)。

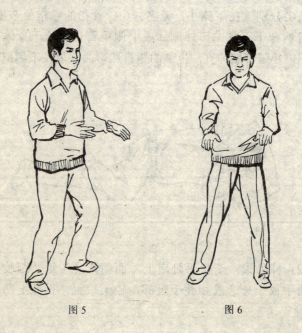

图 5　　　　　图 6

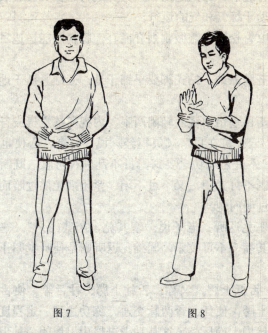

图7　　　　　　图8

2.1.4　锻炼姿势的要领

对于练功姿势的要求《遵生八笺》引《心书》说："厚铺坐褥，宽解衣带，端身直脊，唇齿相着，舌柱上腭，微开其目，常视鼻端。"练功的姿势虽然很多，但其总的要求则是：

(1) 宽解衣带。只有宽解衣带，才能使经络通畅，气不留滞。

(2) 头如顶物。或称为悬顶，就是头要端正，下颌微收，有一种微微上顶之劲，这样颈部才能放松端正。

(3) 沉肩垂肘。就是两肩放松，两肘下垂不可用劲挺紧。

(4) 含胸拔背。就是脊要直，不可随意弯曲，或依靠他物，在脊直的基础上胸要内含。

(5) 舒腰松腹。腰腹是练气、运气的重要部位。腹为练气之炉，腰为肾之府，命门之所在，经脉运行之要关腰腹放松而不懈怠。才有助于练气和气的运行。

(6) 收臀松膝。臀微收则脊能直，膝松则能运达足三阳、足三阴之气。

(7) 五趾抓地。站式脚要平铺于地，五趾紧抓于地，使身体稳如泰山。

(8) 两目垂帘内视。轻闭两眼，内视所练之气或行气之处。《阴府经》云："机在目"，《灵枢经》说："目者，心使也"，"心者，神之舍也"。目为练功之要窍，目不乱则神可收，既断幻觉，又断阳光。既不可紧闭，又不可不闭。紧闭则光黑过暗而昏，不闭则神露，过明而驰。

(9) 塞兑返听。老子说："塞其兑，闭其门户"。塞兑，这里是指轻合其嘴，不可咬牙，紧缩。返听则是使听觉归于自身以断外缘。

(10) 舌抵上腭。又称：舌柱上腭、柱舌等。使舌自然地轻轻上抵于上腭，使任、督两脉交通。练功达到一定程度，舌抵上腭之力自然增大而后缩，这是功夫进展中出现的一种现象，不要故意追求。

(11) 若练导引功，则使推、摩、揉等手法，姿势随手活动，放松，不可僵硬。

2.2 调息

调息又叫呼吸、息法、吐纳等，是气功锻炼的重要一环。古人特别注意呼吸的锻炼，在古代著作中，我们可以看到众多的呼吸锻炼名称，如服气、食气、进气、咽气、行气、采气等。也有很多呼吸的方法，如上息、下息、满息、冲息、持息、长息、深息等。根据我们练功的需要，最常用的有以下几种。

2.2.1 自然呼吸

自然呼吸即一般的生理状态下的呼吸。由于男女生理上的差异及人们习惯的不同,出现的自然呼吸有自然胸式呼吸为主者,有自然腹式呼吸为主者,有自然混合呼吸者,不管哪种均取自然状态,而进行某种有意识的呼吸,此种呼吸是练功者常用的一种呼吸方法。

2.2.2 顺腹式呼吸

是通过自然呼吸的锻炼,逐渐加以意识导引,加强呼吸的腹式运动。其方法是:在吸气时轻轻用意念使腹肌放松,腹部自然隆起,在呼气时,轻轻用意念使腹肌收缩,经过一段时间的锻炼,使腹肌起伏逐渐地、自然地加大,切忌勉强用力。一般锻炼时意守肚脐易于形成顺腹式呼吸。

2.2.3 逆腹式呼吸

逆腹式呼吸,是练气功和发放外气的一种主要呼吸方法。锻炼的方法是:吸气时用意念支配腹肌逐渐收缩,使腹部凹下;呼气时用意念支配腹肌逐渐放松隆起,经过一个时期的锻炼,逆腹式呼吸就成为一种练功过程中的自然的腹式呼吸了。

逆腹式呼吸一般练熟后可以逐渐配合提肛动作,即吸气时肛门微缩,前阴微收,呼气时肛门同时放松。

2.2.4 其它呼吸法

除练以上呼吸方法外,在锻炼方法上还可以练吸长呼短、吸短呼长、鼻呼鼻吸、鼻吸口呼、呼后停闭、吸后停闭等,这要根据练功的不同方法和练功之不同阶段配合锻炼。在讲到具体功法时再详细介绍。

2.2.5 锻炼呼吸的要领

(1) 练动功、导引功或静功开始时主要练姿势，使姿势动作熟炼、放松后，再配合练呼吸，否则易导致呼吸紧迫，情绪紧张，胸闷，头痛等。

(2) 呼吸最后达到的要求是深、长、匀、细。这是呼吸功夫的积累所形成的，不可故意拉长、硬压。

(3) 练导引功，手法的动作多配合呼吸，如顺手三阴经向指端推为呼；顺手三阳经向肩、头部推为吸，这是根据经络的走向规定的。经络的走行方向是：手三阴经从胸走手，手三阳经从手走头，足三阴经从足走胸腹，足三阳经从头走足。

(4) 在练呼吸之前最好先开口呼气，意想身中百脉不通处，体内之浊气，均随息出，后闭口纳清，共三次。然后任其自然，慢慢用意念调整所要练的呼吸方法。

2.3 调心

调心，又叫意念、心法。意念的锻炼是气功锻炼最重要的一环。《摄生三要》说："聚精在于养气，养气在于存神。神之于气，犹母之于子也。故神凝则气聚，神散则气消，若保惜精气，而不知存神，是茹其华而忘其根矣。"因为心藏神，所以这里说的存神就是指调心。他强调了在练功中精气神的关系，并说明其中神所居的重要地位。

1. 在练功中意念集中于自身某一部或穴位上。如上丹田、下丹田、中丹田、涌泉、内劳宫、指端、手掌等，或集中于身外的某一物或某一静止不动的点上叫定位性意守。

2. 在练功中意念随手法运行，或随气在经络中运行，或意守两手或身体某部位所感应而出现的气感现象，叫定向性意念。

3. 在练功中意念在随呼吸而数息，或某一节律性振动或缓慢的运动，如振桩中的细微振动等，叫节律性意念。

4. 在练功中意想力大，就象真有想象的那样大一样，如意想推山，托天门，拉九牛尾等，叫壮力性意念。

5. 在练功中配合语言诱导活动的一种意念锻炼，如默念字句，意想练功所达到之目的，叫暗示性意念。

6. 在练功中提出一种假借现象，经锻炼可出现一种气的感应，如抚球、按气、贯气、排病气、气热如火、气寒如冰、其气利如剑、其气柔如棉等，叫假借性意念。

7. 意念锻炼的要领

(1) 意念的活动要自然地与呼吸、姿势相配合，如在动功或导引功中，意念要配合姿势、手法升、降、开、合的运动。

(2) 意念活动要做到自然，在入静的状态下逐渐进行锻炼。

(3) 练意要有一个"信"字，不管是哪种意念活动都坚信通过锻炼，能达到其目的，但不急于求成。

(4) 意念中出现景象不喜不恐、不虑不言。

2.4 常用穴窍

气功疗法常意守某些穴位来练气或运气，也常自我按摩某些穴位来激发、调理气机，以达到治病的目的。兹将常用穴窍介绍如下。

1. **百会**。在两耳尖直上，头顶中央是穴。

穴在人体至高正中处，是手足三阳经与督脉之会穴，故曰诸阳之会。自我按摩此穴可治头痛、头晕、目眩、健忘、脱肛、子宫下垂等症。

2. **印堂**。在两眉之间。此穴为神识之穴，主治头痛，头晕及神识之病。

3. **上丹田**。又称泥丸宫，在印堂内3寸。本穴为练气功的要穴，乃藏神练气之所，练气功意守上丹田能强神益智，但初练一般不意守上丹田。

4. **太阳**。在目外眦与眉梢外陷凹处。自我按摩导引此穴可治头痛、感冒等病。

5. **鼻准**。在鼻头之端。揉按此穴可治鼻塞流涕。

6. **风府**。在项后入发际一寸处。凡疾病因之风者，气者均可自我按摩此处。

7. **风池**。在风府两侧，项肌外缘凹陷处，自我按摩导引此处可治感冒、头痛、目赤肿痛。

8. **玉枕关**。在枕骨粗隆下，风府上方。为练气通督脉之要穴。

9. **血浪**。在项部两侧胸锁乳突肌前缘处。自我推揉此穴可降血压、治头晕、目眩等。

10. **缺盆**。在乳头直上锁骨上缘凹陷中。自我按摩此穴可以调肺、胃之气、治疗咳嗽、胸闷、气喘等。

11. **膻中**。在两乳之中间。中丹田即在此穴内3寸处，是气之会穴，故自我按摩此处能治一切气分之病。

12. **中脘**。在肚脐与剑突之间。自我按摩导引此穴是治疗腹胀、腹痛、胸闷、厌食诸症的要穴。

13. **神阙**。在肚脐处，此穴为后天之气舍及先天之气之所存，故自我按摩导引此穴可兼治先后天之病。

14. **关元**。在脐下3寸处。本穴又有丹田之称，练气功多意守此处，是练气积气治疗先天元气不足之症的要穴。

15. **下丹田**。在脐下1.3寸，向内3寸处，是练静功意守的常用穴位，也是气机发动感觉明显的地方。

16. **会阴**。在两阴之间。是任、督、冲三脉之所起，练功时往往会阴穴跳动，是气机发动的现象。

17. **肩井**。在肩上凹陷处。自我按摩导引此穴可以通调周身之气机，疏通诸经之经气，是治疗项痛，手臂痛，下肢痛的要穴。

18. **命门**。在第二、三腰椎之间是治疗命门火衰、阳萎、白浊、腰痛等症的要穴。

19. **长强**。又称尾闾关，在尾闾骨端下陷中，以意运周天功起自尾闾关，是练功导气的主要穴位。

20. **三关**。是指练功，气通督脉时的三个重要穴位，有尾闾关、夹脊关、玉枕关。尾闾关，即长强处；夹脊关，在命门之两侧；玉枕关，在枕骨粗隆下入脑处。

21. **曲池**。屈肘时，当肘横纹外端处，自我按摩导引此穴可治感冒、头痛、鼻塞等。

22. **合谷**。在手背第一、二掌骨之间。主治头痛、牙痛、耳痛、感冒等。

23. **内劳宫**。在手掌心中点处。此穴是调气要穴，练导引功时，注意体会此处之气感。

24. **足三里**。在外膝眼下3寸处。本穴是保健和治疗腹痛、腹胀、下肢冷痛等病的要穴。

25. **涌泉**。在足底足趾蹠屈时呈凹陷处。本穴能引火归原，是练气和导引按摩的要穴。

2.5 练功中应注意的问题

1. 练功首先要将自己所练功法中的动作、呼吸、意念、要领弄清楚、将手法、穴位选好、找准、经过一段学习、较熟练了，就可以坚持锻炼。

2. 要充分发挥自己的主动性，有信心，有决心，有恒心，循序渐进地进行认真锻炼。练功前要将自己的工作、学习、生活等各方面的事情都安排好，不要带着思想问题和紧张不安的情绪来练功。

3. 一般要选择空气新鲜、环境安静的地方练功，在室内练功也要注意安静和空气流通，但不宜在迎风或风扇下练功。

4. 练功前要做好准备工作，首先要情绪安定下来，解好大小便，放松腰带，取下手表、眼镜，以免影响气机和血液循环。有些导引手法需暴露体表，有些具体的功法要严格遵守其要领和注意事项。

5. 练功次数，有些导引的动作次数，最好按要求练。但练功总时间的长短，也要根据自己的体质、病情和练功的进度灵活掌握，不可勉强延长时间和增加次数，应留有余力，留有余兴，以不感到疲劳为度。

6. 不要在过饱或过饥饿时练功。一般要在进餐一个小时以后再练功。

7. 以气功治疗疾病时，可以同时配合药物或其他治疗方法进行综合治疗。妇女月经期练功时不宜过长。不要向下体引导过多的意念活动。

8. 练功中体内出现热、胀、酸、痛、麻、痒、凉、虫爬、肌肉跳动等感觉，这是体内气机发动的现象，不要惊恐紧张，也不要好奇追求，一切顺其自然。

9. 练功中要节制房事，对烟、酒、茶及辛辣之物都适当控制，逐渐戒烟。

10. 练功中突然受到惊恐，如大的响声，或别人意外骚扰，或练功中出现奇特现象，都不要紧张、害怕，要找出原因，使情绪安定下来再练功。

11. 练功要做到起功稳，练功稳，收功稳。不可草草起功和收功，以免气不归原或气机紊乱。

12. 发放外气治病者，要经过练气、导气、发功治疗等学习和锻炼，达到发功的要求时，方可给人治病，详见第四章。

3 功　　法

3.1 放松功

　　放松功是静功的一种比较容易掌握的基础功法。不管练静功还是练动功，首先要做到松静自然，做到放松。所以放松功可以作为初学气功者的入门锻炼功法。

功法

　　1. 姿势：站式、坐式或卧式均可，不管选用那种姿势，都要做到松静自然，全身肌肉、脏腑组织及精神尽可能地放松，两眼轻闭，亦可微睁双眼。

　　2. 三线放松法：是将人体分为三条线。第一条线是头、颈、肩，上肢的两侧面；第二条线是面、颈、胸、腹及两下肢的前面；第三条线是头、颈、背、腰及两下肢的后面。

　　在练功时，注意一个部位，然后默念"松"字，再注意次一个部位默念"松"字，从上到下，自第一条线开始，逐次放松完三条线，然后再循环回来锻炼，一般3～5个循环即可。自然呼吸。

　　3. 部位放松法：是按部位自上而下，先注意一个部位，再默念"松"字，从头到肩、上肢、背、腰、髋、两下肢逐次放松，3～5个循环。自然呼吸。

　　4. 整体放松法：就整个身体做为一个整体，象洗温水淋浴似的，先从头开始，水平地向下缓缓放松。自然呼吸。

　　5. 收功：做完放松锻炼后一般不再默念"松"字，静静地按原式练一会，即可搓搓脸，搓搓手而收功，亦可两手相叠（男左手在下，女右手在下），按在脐部，先顺时针方向从小圈转至腹侧共 36 圈，再反方向转 36 圈至脐，再搓脸，搓手收功。

应用

1. 用作保健或初学气功者的基础功法，也可用以治疗各种慢性疾病，如高血压病、神经官能症、支气管炎、支气管哮喘、更年期综合症、胃炎、胃及十二指肠溃疡、慢性盆腔炎和诱导睡眠等。

2. 高血压、头痛、头晕等症，多用三线放松法，并配合头面功锻炼。

3. 肺、胃、心等部位的疾患用部位放松法，并重点放松有病的部位。

注意事项

1. 每天可练 1～4 次，一般根据自己的情况选炼一种放松功。

2. 各种放松一般用自然呼吸，也可以与意念结合起来，一般是吸气时注意部位，呼气时默念"松"字。

3. 注意部位时要轻轻的似想到该处，又似未想到该处。初练杂念经常出现，是自然现象。

4. 保持情绪轻松愉快，愤怒或过于兴奋时不宜练功。

5. 如卧式出现昏睡时，可改练坐式或站式。

3.2 内养功

内养功是以默念字句与呼吸相结合的锻炼方法，它对促进消化系统和呼吸系统的功能均有很好的作用。

功法

1. 鼻吸鼻呼法：卧位或坐位，选用顺腹式呼吸或逆腹式呼吸。用鼻吸气时,舌抵上腭,引气到小腹丹田部(脐下1.3寸),默想"自"字,然后停顿呼吸,默想"己"或"己静"或"己静坐身体"或"己静坐身体能健";最后呼气时舌放下,默念"静"、"坐"、"好"、"康",即成为"自己静"、"自己静坐"、"自己静坐身体好"、"自己静坐身体能健康"等字句。先从字少的字句练起,最多亦不超过九个字,其中第一字为吸气,最后一字为呼气,中间的字为停闭呼吸。

2. 口鼻呼吸法:运用腹式呼吸,吸气时以鼻自然地吸入,引至丹田,随即将气自然从口呼出,然后舌抵上腭,停顿呼吸默念字句。等念完字句,再行吸气。如此周而复始地进行。

3. 收功方法:参照放松功。

应用

防治慢性胃炎、胃溃疡、十二指肠溃疡、慢性肝炎、神经衰弱、高血压、月经不调、痛经等症。

注意事项

1. 每天练功1~4次,每次10~60分钟。
2. 初练时用顺腹式呼吸,待熟练后,改为逆腹式呼吸。停闭呼吸,一定先从三个字开始练,逐渐增多,切不可强"停闭呼吸"或用力鼓腹。
3. 久练小腹部有温热感,是正常现象。

3.3 强壮功

强壮功是通过呼吸及意守丹田的锻炼,使内气强盛的功法,有健身与防治疾病的作用。

功法

1. 自然呼吸法：盘坐式或站式，应用自然呼吸，但要注意呼吸逐渐达到均匀、细缓。同时，注意意守丹田，要似有似无的想，不可过于紧张。

2. 深呼吸法：盘坐式或站式，在练自然呼吸的基础上，呼吸逐渐放慢加长，做到静细、深长、均匀，仍然意守丹田。

3. 逆呼吸法：盘坐式或站式，用逆腹式呼吸，意守丹田。吸气时收腹提肛，气注丹田；呼气时鼓腹，气沉丹田。

应用

用于保健和治疗高血压、神经衰弱、神经官能症、冠心病、关节炎等病症。

注意事项

1. 每日练 1~4 次，每次 10~60 分钟。
2. 呼吸细、匀、深、长是经过长期锻炼形成的，不可强求或故意憋气。每次练功以不疲劳为度。

3.4 头面功

头面功，是调整面部经络穴位，促进气血运行的功法，有健美、保健、祛病、防病的作用。

功法

1. 预备：正坐或站位，全身放松，排除杂念，舌抵上腭，两目微闭。

2. 推前额：两手食、中、无名指并拢，用指面从两眉中点向前发际直推 24~50 次，然后再自前额中点向两侧分推 24~50 次（见图 9）。用匀细长呼吸，呼气时用力推，吸气时略轻，注意手下之气感。

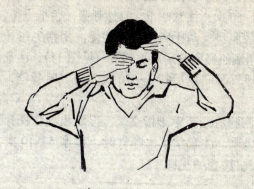

图 9

3. 揉运太阳：以两手中指按眉后陷凹处，向耳后方向旋揉 24～50 次（见图 10）。意念与呼吸同上。

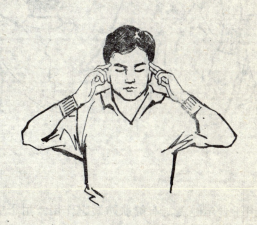

图 10

4. 浴面：用两手掌从额上向两侧，再向下搓摩，然后以鼻两侧反转向上搓摩 24～50 次，再向反方向搓摩 24～50 次，自然呼吸，注意两手掌下。

5. 梳发：两手五指自然分开微屈，象梳发一样从前向后顺理梳发 24～50 次。注意掌下，自然呼吸，舌抵上腭。

6. 扫散胆经：两手四指微屈并拢，用指尖在耳上，头之侧面，以额角顺胆经向脑后摩擦扫散（见图 11）。注意掌下，用匀长呼吸，呼气时向脑后扫 5～10 次，吸气时暂停，共做 5～10 息。

7. 搓摩脑后：两手十指交叉，以掌根抱住枕骨下部，从上向后下方搓摩，注意掌下，呼气时，搓摩 5～10 次，吸气时暂停，共做 5～10 息（见图 12）。

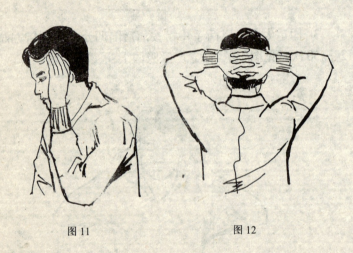

图 11　　　　　　图 12

应用

1. 适用于青年健美，有健肤防皱之作用。用于中老年人保健或防治脱发、高血压、面瘫、头痛、头晕、感冒、偏头痛等症。

2. 健美者，多做浴面、推前额、梳发三项功法。自然呼吸，注意手法的感应，并意想经过保健皱纹已消，气血通畅等美的形象。

3. 高血压、神经衰弱等头痛、头晕者,多做扫散胆经、运太阳、搓摩脑后。意注手下。呼气时用推摩的手法,导引气机下行。吸气时暂停,但不可憋气,或用暴力搓摩。

注意事项

1. 每天练功 1~4 次,每个手法操作的次数可根据自己的情况,逐渐增多,用力逐渐增大。

2. 要注意修养性格,不可大怒或用脑过度,生活起居要有规律。若脑力劳动后,头晕不适,即可练一遍,能消除疲劳。

3.5 眼功

眼功是以锻炼眼睛为主的功法,有调节肝经气脉,疏肝明目的作用。

功法

1. 预备:正坐或站位,全身放松,排除杂念,两目平视。

2. 八字运目:意想气在眼眶内运转,眼球亦随之转动,先从左侧睛明穴起,沿左眼眶上缘,向外至眼外角;再向内沿眶下缘,转至右眼睛明穴,再沿右眼眶上缘,转至眶下缘,行"∞"字,回至左睛明处,共 8 次。然后从右睛明穴起,向反方向转 8 次。自然呼吸,以意领气,气行意到。

3. 按目运气:两拇指按眼眶内上角(上睛明),意念集中于此处,吸气时两拇指向眼眶及眼后方按压;呼气时,两拇指轻挤眼球。以眼内轻微酸胀为度,共 8 次(见图 13)。

4. 浴目:轻闭双眼,用两手四指指面,相互擦热,然后在眼内角向外擦 24 次(见图 14)。自然呼吸,意注手下。

应用

1. 适用于眼睛的保健及青少年近视、远视、散光的预防和治疗。有调整肝经气脉,疏肝明目的作用。若能与疏肝明目功配合锻炼则效果更佳。

2. 适用于中老年人头晕眼花、视物模糊、眼干涩、目赤肿痛、眼肌疲劳等。

3. 练完功后,最好轻闭双眼,稍微休息一会儿。

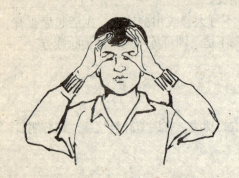
图 13

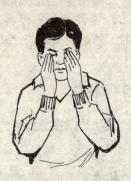
图 14

注意事项

1. 每天练功 1~4 次。看书写字眼睛疲劳时,可选练第 1,3 两节,能消除疲劳,保护视力。

2. 注意不要在光线暗淡的地方看书,如眼睛有近视、散光、花眼等病,要及时配镜子,注意眼睛卫生,防止眼睛疲劳。

3.6 鼻齿功

鼻齿功是宣通鼻窍,固齿防龋的功法。

功法

1. 预备:坐位或站位,排除鼻涕、松静自然,调匀呼吸。

2. 洗皂：用两手大拇指背，相互搓热。然后，轻轻上下摩擦鼻之两侧，吸气时搓擦 5 次，呼气时搓擦 5 次，共 6 息（见图 15）。

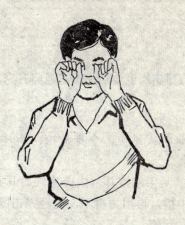

图 15

3. 揉鼻端：以右手中指端按鼻尖部，一吸气左转 5 次，一呼气右转 5 次，共 6 息。

4. 叩齿与咬牙固气：上下牙齿相互叩击 36 次，然后咽津液。每天于大小便时，闭口咬牙至大小便解完。慢慢放松，自然呼吸，意存牙齿部位，以固元气。

应用

1. 鼻齿功，有宣通鼻窍，固齿防龋的功能，叩齿咬牙固气一节，最好形成练功习惯，久练必有好处。

2. 适用于健康人保健，可以防治鼻塞、鼻流浊涕、感冒、牙痛、龋齿等。注意手法导引与呼吸意念的配合。

注意事项

1. 一般每天练 1～2 次。防治鼻炎，可选做洗皂一节，每天练 2~4 次。

2. 用力要柔和深透，不可用蛮力，或损伤皮肤。
3. 注意口腔卫生，练功前排净鼻涕。

3.7 耳功

耳功是防治耳病的主要功夫，有通经开窍之作用。

功法

1. 预备：坐位或站位，全身放松，两耳反听，闭口垂帘，自然呼吸，排除杂念。
2. 鸣天鼓：两手掌按耳（内劳宫穴对耳孔）手指放于脑后部，用食指压中指，再用力滑下，轻轻弹击脑后部 24 次。自己可以听到咚咚的声音。
3. 按耳导气：两手掌紧按两耳孔，再放开，使内"耳"鼓气 10 次。按压放开时不可用力过大过猛，既要紧按速放，又要轻柔适中。
4. 按摩耳轮：用拇、食指轻捏耳轮之上部，顺耳轮自上而下反复按摩 24 次。使耳轮有热感为好。

应用

1. 本功有通窍之作用，适用于保健，预防耳病。
2. 治疗耳鸣、耳聋、耳痛等症时可配合补肾的功法，如服黑气法，搓腰肾，搓涌泉等，效果更好。

注意事项

1. 保健者每天练 1~2 次，治疗疾病每天练 2~4 次，不可用力过大，特别是放开时。
2. 注意耳内卫生，时常反听内养。若耳鸣者，可用两掌轻搓耳部，微微活动一下头部，再行此功。

3.8 颈项功

颈项功是防治颈部疾病的功法，有舒筋活络，滑利关节之作用。

功法

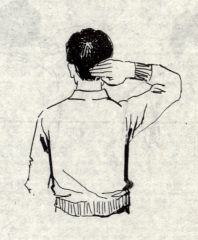

图16

1. 预备：站位或坐位，颈部放松，自然呼吸，两目平视。
2. 疏导风池：以两手拇指按风池，吸气时轻揉5次，呼气时轻揉5次，共14息；然后以两手拇、食、中指捏齐，轻轻叩击此穴30次。
3. 推导天柱：头微低，用右手（或左手）四指面在颈后正中，呼气时从上向下推7次；吸气时暂停，共做8息（见图16）。
4. 推导血浪：右手四指并拢，用指面推导颈侧血浪部。呼气时，先在颈部左侧（男先左侧，女先右侧），从颌下顺胸锁乳突肌推抹至锁骨处，吸气时暂停，共 14 息（见图 17）。然后推右侧。

5. 转颈导气：吸气时头颈从左前转至后，呼气时从后转向前逆时针方向转。然后再反方向转，各 8 次。

6. 两手与颈项争力：两手十指交叉，抱后颈部，吸气时两手向前拉，同时头微仰，向后用力仰视，呼气时放松，共 9 息（见图 18）。

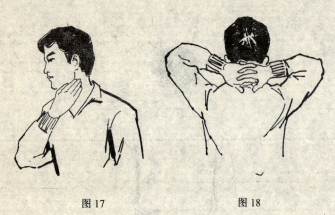

图 17　　　　　　　图 18

应用

1. 适用于保健以及治疗颈项疼痛、颈椎病、落枕、颈肌纤维炎等。
2. 高血压、头痛、头目眩晕者，重点练揉风池、推导血浪，再配合头面功之扫散、梳发、以及放松功等锻炼。
3. 颈椎病、落枕等，多练转颈导气、推导天柱、两手与颈项争力等节。

注意事项

1. 每天练 1～4 次。最好早晨要保持练功 1 次。
2. 练功时用力与动作要协调，活动范围和力量要逐渐增大,不可速度过快,要与呼吸密切配合。

3. 避免高枕或长时间低头。屈颈工作者,当劳累时,要选练本功中几节,以舒筋活络,滑利关节,解除疲劳。

3.9 肩臂功

肩臂功是防治肩臂部疾病的功法,有通行手三阴、三阳经气血,消肿止痛,滑利关节之作用。

功法

1. 预备:坐位或站位。排除杂念,全身放松,自然呼吸。
2. 捶击肩臂:先以左手握空拳,从右肩外侧轻击至手腕3～5遍;再以同法从上至下捶击上肢内侧,前侧各3～5遍。然后,用右手以同法捶击左上肢内侧、外侧、前侧各3～5遍。

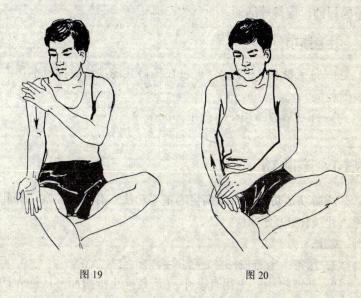

图19　　　　　　图20

3. 通导手三阴三阳经:坐位,右手仰掌放于右腿上,以左手掌从右肩内侧顺手三阴经向下推摩至手掌（见图19），边推边慢慢呼气，意念随手掌下行。然后右手变俯掌，左手掌转至右手背，顺手三阳经推摩至肩部，向上推摩时吸气，意念随掌运行，共7次。再以左手按摩合谷穴36次，不可憋气，两上肢力求放松（见图20）。然后再以同法通导左上肢手三阴手三阳经。

4. 按揉曲池：用左手拇指按右曲池穴，按揉36次，然后以右手拇指按揉左手曲池穴36次。

5. 按揉合谷：以左手拇指按揉右手合谷穴36次，再以右手按揉左手合谷穴36次。

应用

1. 本功有通行手三阴、三阳经气血，消肿止痛，滑利关节之作用。用于保健以及治疗肩臂酸痛麻木、扭伤、四肢无力等。

2. 若肩臂痛，除练以上功法外，可以配合练肩、肘、腕关节的屈伸，旋转等活动。

注意事项

1. 每天练功1~2次，也可在练习其他功法后再行本功，以调理经气。

2. 练功后暂不用冷水洗手、洗澡等。

3.10 胸胁功

胸胁功是防治胸胁部病症的主要功法。有宽胸理气，舒肝降逆，止咳化痰的作用。

功法

1. 预备：坐势或站势，呼吸调匀，全身放松。

2. 推理膻中：先用食、中、无名、小指指面，从胸骨切迹下推至剑突36次，自然呼吸，意注指下。

3. 推导理气：呼气时，以右手掌自胸部中线向左侧推 5~10 次，吸气时暂停，共 10 息。再以左手掌自胸部中线向右推 10 息，意随手动。

4. 摩胁降气：呼气时以两手平掌、从两腋下搓摩至腹侧 5~10 次。

应用

1. 用于保健以及防治胸闷、胸痛、呼吸不利、痰多，气喘等。

2. 治疗哮喘、支气管炎等病，要配合理肺功或呬字诀进行锻炼。

注意事项

1. 每天练 1~2 次，也可练完其他功法以后练本功，以作为收功或辅助功法。

2. 练功时，呼吸细缓均匀自然，不可憋气，肌肉放松。

3. 最好选择空气新鲜的环境练功，按顺序将三节做完。

3.11 腹部功

腹部功是防治消化系统疾病的常用功法。有健脾益气，和胃调中的作用。

功法

1. 预备：仰卧位，全身放松，舌抵上腭，自然呼吸。

2. 揉腹壮气：以右手按放于中脘穴处，自右向左旋揉 36 次，再在脐部左右旋揉 36 次。

3. 分腹消食：呼气时，以两手四指或全掌在腹部中线自剑突向耻骨联合推 36 次，再从剑突向两侧斜下分推 36 次，意念注意手下推摩的感觉。

4. 揉丹壮气：左手在下右手叠压在左手上，旋揉小腹中点36次；然后再以五指捏拢，轻轻叩击 50～100 次。

应用

1. 用于保健和防治腹痛、腹胀、腹泻、便秘、厌食以及结肠炎、胃炎、胃溃疡、十二指肠溃疡等消化系统病症。

2. 若腹泻、便秘者，先练周天自转功，然后再练本功，可提高疗效。

3. 治疗溃疡病、结肠炎等，最好先练内养功或强壮功，然后练本功法。

注意事项

1. 保健者，每天练 1～2 次，治病者练 2～4 次。

2. 练功前要解除大、小便，最好饭后 1 小时后再练功，饥饿时也不宜练功。

3. 手法不宜快，要与呼吸、意念相配合，轻重适宜，不能蛮压或暴力推摩。

3.12 腰部功

腰部功是腰部保健的功法，有强筋壮骨、健腰益肾的作用。

功法

1. 预备：站位，全身放松，自然呼吸。

2. 运腰强筋：两手叉腰，以腰部为轴，向左旋转 36 圈，再向右旋

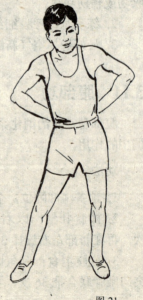

图21

转 36 圈（见图 21）。

3. 捶腰骶：以双手握空拳交互捶击腰两侧肾区及骶部各 36 次。

4. 两手掌搓热自上向下搓摩腰部及两肾区，到温热为止。

应用

1. 用于保健和防治腰痛、腰酸、膝软等。
2. 肾虚腰痛者，多与回春功、铁裆功等配合锻炼。

注意事项

1. 每日练功 1～2 次。
2. 节制房事，在练过其他功法后，可再练此功法，以加强腰部的锻炼。

3.13 下肢功

下肢功是强健腰腿，防治下肢部疾病的功法，有舒筋活络的作用。

功法

1. 预备：坐位。
2. 拍击下肢：一腿微屈，一腿伸直，两手自然张开，以掌根用力，轻轻拍击伸直侧下肢，从大腿根至小腿部 3～5 遍，再以同法拍击另一侧。
3. 通导足三阴、三阳经：坐于床上，左手放于右大腿根的前面，右手在右腿根外后侧，顺足三阳经向下推摩至足部。向下推时呼气，意随掌行（见图 22）。然后两手反转向足内侧，顺足三阴经推摩至大腿根部。向上推摩时吸气，意随掌行。共 7～9 遍（见图 23）。

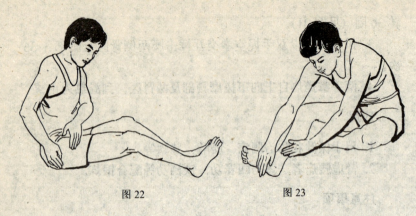

图 22　　　　　图 23

应用

本功法有通行足三阴、三阳之气血，强健腰腿，祛风散寒之作用。

1. 用于保健，防治坐骨神经痛、关节炎。
2. 防治寒湿腿膝疼痛，软弱无力、下肢麻木，解除疲劳等。可以配合练鹤翔庄功，或自发动功。

注意事项

1. 保健者，每天练 1～2 次。防治疾病可练 2～4 次。劳累后即可锻炼几次，能消除疲劳。
2. 练功时最好穿短裤。

3.14　理心功

理心功，是调理心经气脉的功法。有补心安神，活血通经的作用。

功法

1. 服赤气法

(1) 预备：站位、坐位或卧位，全身放松，自然呼吸，排除杂念。

(2) 先叩齿36次，舌搅津液于口内，并将津液分三次咽下，意念随之，送入丹田。

(3) 再意想赤红之气，并以鼻吸之，吸之满口，呼气时慢慢送至心脏，再送至丹田，使心肾相交，通调周身，做7次或14次。然后还原至预备式收功。

2. 摩胸呵气法

(1) 预备：姿势同上。

(2) 如服赤气法，先叩齿，搅舌，咽津毕，右手平掌放于胸部心前区，慢慢吸气，再缓缓呼气，口念"呵"字诀，意念存于掌下，共6～12息（见图24），同时手掌向顺时针方向轻摩。

3. 理心导气法

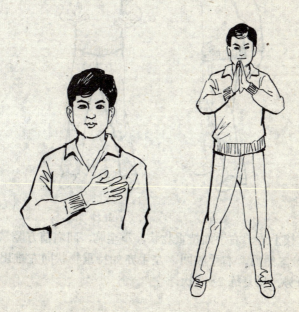

图24　　　　　图25

（1）站位或坐位，全身放松，自然呼吸，舌抵上腭。先在胸前轻合两手（见图25），静站片刻，意想丹田。

（2）接上势，两手转掌向外，两臂顺身体两侧分推至背后（见图26），静止片刻。

（3）接上势，两手翻掌向上，提至胸部两侧（见图27）。

（4）接上势，两手慢慢平伸向前，劲在中指端，手掌外翻大鱼际处微下压（见图28）。

（5）接上势，两手握拳似拉重物状，沿身体两侧拉向背后（见图29）。

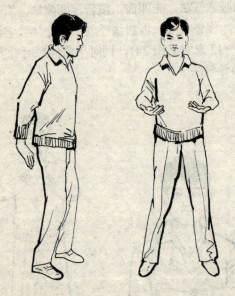

图26　　　　图27

（6）接上势，右手如持重物状，举至胸，向右前方竖掌推出（见图30）。然后，右手收回，左手亦如持重物状向左推出，最后恢复原势。反复练2～3次。

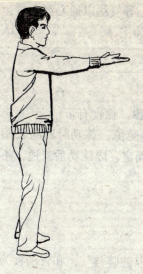
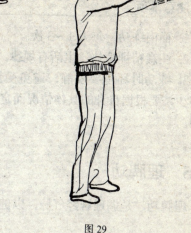

图 28　　　　　图 29

应用

1. 用于防治心悸、怔忡、心痛、失眠等症。如冠心病、高血压、心律失常、风湿性心脏病、心脏神经官能症等。

2. 身体虚弱者可采用坐位或卧位。

3. 虚症患者，宜练服赤气法，有补心益气安神养血的作用。亦可配合理心导气法，有通经络的作用。心力衰竭者，以养为主，配合内养功锻炼，意念只守丹田。

4. 实症患者，宜练摩胸呵气

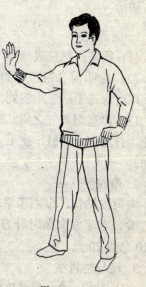

图 30

法，以泻实祛痰为主，再配合理心导气法以通心经之气。

5. 保健者，以练摩胸呵气法为主。

注意事项

1. 面南练功，每天 1~3 次。
2. 注意精神愉快，生活有规律，饮食有节。
3. 练功时环境要安静，避免受惊，练功时间的长短、次数的多少，要根据自身的具体情况而定，以练功后舒适、不疲劳为原则。

3.15 理脾功

理脾功，是调理脾经气脉，以健脾益气、和胃消食为主的功法。

功法

1. 服黄气法

(1) 预备：站位或坐位。全身放松，自然呼吸，排除杂念。

(2) 先叩齿 36 次，舌搅津液于口内，并将津液分 3 次咽下，用意念送至脐上中脘处。

(3) 再意想黄气之象，吸气时令其满口，呼气时慢慢送至中脘处，并通融于四肢、皮毛，如此 5~10 次。然后还原至预备式收功。

2. 摩脘呼气法

坐位或站位，以右手掌轻轻平放于上腹中脘部，慢慢呼气。呼气时，右手掌向顺时针方向摩（见图 31），同时念"呼"字诀，做 10 息或 20 息。

3. 疏导脾胃法

(1) 站位。全身自然放松，呼吸自然，以腰为轴，带动两臂左右摇摆（见图32）。向左摇目观左，向右摇目观右，意至足跟。

（2）跪坐，两手掌平按于床上，入静片刻，上身前俯，臀部抬起，向左回头作虎视状，目视远方（见图33），再向右回头虎视。左右各5次。

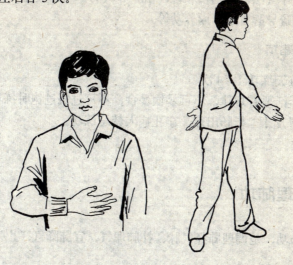

图 31　　　　图 32

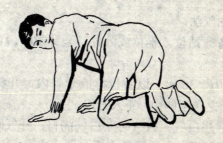

图 33

应用

1. 用于保健及预防腹胀、腹泻、便秘等。

2. 用于治疗慢性胃炎及十二指肠溃疡、结肠炎、胃肠官能症等。配合腹部功法锻炼效果更佳。

3. 脾胃虚寒症，宜练服黄气法，有健脾益气的作用；实热症练摩脘呼气法，有消食和胃，祛除邪气的作用。虚症与实症均可配合练疏导脾胃法、内养功等。

注意事项

1. 每天练功1～4次。
2. 生活要有规律，不可暴饮暴食，不可过饥过饱时练功。
3. 胃及十二指肠出血、穿孔病人禁忌练功。

3.16 理肺功

理肺功，是调理肺经气脉、补肺理气、宣肺降气、止咳化痰的功法。

功法

1. 服白气法

(1)预备：站位、坐位或卧位，全身放松，自然呼吸，排除杂念。

(2)先叩齿36次，以舌搅津液于口内，并将津液分3次咽下，意念随之送至胸中，下入丹田。

(3)再意想白气，吸气时令白气满口，呼气时将气慢慢送至两肺，下至丹田，充入周身皮毛。做9次或18次，然后还原至预备式收功。

2. 摩胸呬气法

站位或坐位。两手掌分别平放于胸部两侧，慢慢吸气。呼气时，口念呬字诀,同时两手掌旋摩胸部(见图34),摩6息至12息。

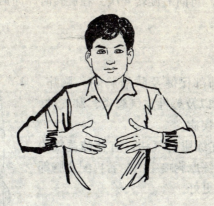

图 34

3. 理肺导气法

(1) 弓背呼吸:自然盘坐,两手掌柱地,挺胸吸满气,略停片刻(见图35),再弓背缩胸,同时呼气(见图36),做4～9次。

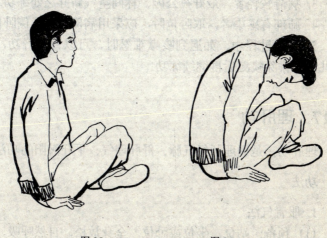

图 35　　　　图 36

(2) 理肺内外转：站位并膝，两手掌扶膝上，先向左旋转 4 次（见图 37），再向右旋转 4 次。在旋转时，向后旋时吸气，向前旋时呼气。

应用

1. 用于肺部保健及防治胸闷、胸痛、气喘、痰多，以及慢性支气管炎、肺气肿、支气管哮喘等疾病。
2. 虚症宜练服白气法，有补肺益气的作用。实症宜练摩胸呬字法。若再配合胸部功锻炼则效果更好。

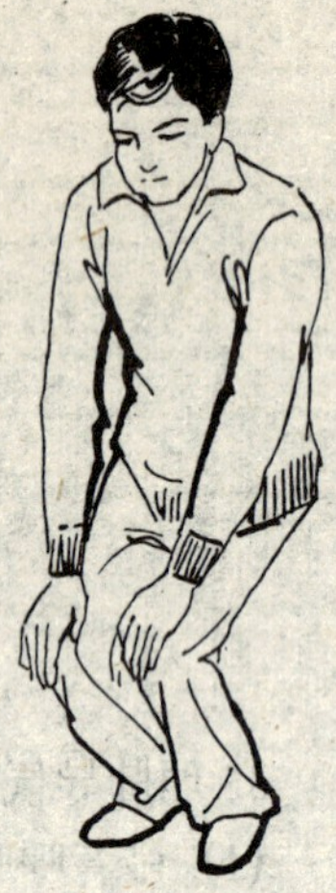

注意事项

1. 每天练功 2～4 次。每次 10～40 分钟。
2. 练功期间禁忌吸烟、喝酒、吃生冷食物等。
3. 病情较轻者，最好在公园、林间空气新鲜之处练功。
4. 肺部有感染者，取卧位时，应采用病侧在下的侧卧位。
5. 练功过程中，如遇到咳嗽难忍时，可以暂不行功，先咳嗽几声，排除痰涎后再继续练功。

图 37

3.17 理肝功

理肝功，是调理肝经气脉、舒肝理气、平肝潜阳的功法。

功法

1. 服青气法
(1) 预备：站位、坐位或卧位。全身放松，自然呼吸，排除杂念，舌抵上腭。

(2) 先叩齿 36 次，舌搅津液，分 3 次咽下，送入两胁，再下归丹田。

(3) 再意想青气、以鼻吸之令满口，呼气时，将气慢慢送至两胁，再下归丹田，做 8 次或 16 次，然后还原至预备式收功。

2. 摩胁嘘气法

站位或坐位，两手掌平放于两胁下，慢慢吸气。呼气时，口念"嘘"字诀，同时两掌轻轻旋摩两胁部（见图 38）。做 10 息或 20 息。

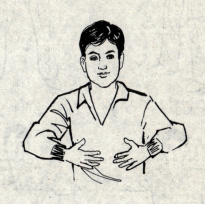

图 38

3. 舒肝导气法

(1) 松静站立，两臂自然下垂，掌心向下，五指微翘，微用力下按，并意想气达手心，直至五指尖，下按 3 次（见图 39）。

(2) 接上势，两手顺势提至胸前两侧，掌心向前（见图 40）意存两掌，向前推出，再收到胸前。

(3) 接上势，两手左右平伸，如鸟舒翼，十指上翘，掌心向左右平推（见图 41），行气至掌心，直至指尖，推 3 次。

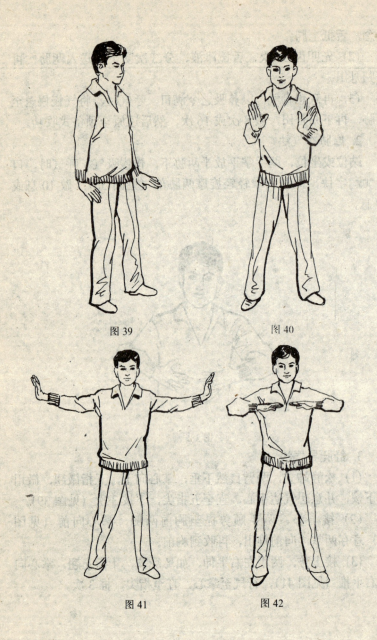

图 39　　　　　图 40

图 41　　　　　图 42

· 308 ·

(4) 接上势，两掌顺势收至胸前，掌心向上，指尖相对，意存两掌，再翻掌向下（见图42），推至耻骨联合处，气行至下丹田，再仰掌托气至中丹田（膻中处），如此3次。然后两手放在体两侧，收功。

应用

1. 用于保健及防治头晕、目眩、口苦咽干、胸胁胀闷等症，适用于高血压、神经官能症、慢性肝炎、胆囊炎、肝脾肿大等病。
2. 肝胆实症宜练摩胁嘘气法，虚症宜练服青气法。虚、实症均可配合练舒肝导气法。

注意事项

1. 每天练功1~4次。
2. 练功期间不可生气，要保持精神愉快。
3. 高血压患者，应配合练放松功、扫散胆经法、推抹血浪等头颈部功法。

3.18 理肾功

理肾功，是疏导肾经气脉、以滋肾壮阳、增补元气的功法。

功法

1. 服黑气法

(1) 预备：站位、坐位或卧位，全身放松，排除杂念，舌抵上腭。

(2) 先叩齿36次，舌搅津液令满口，并将津液分3次咽下，意念随之，送入丹田。

(3) 再意想黑气，以鼻吸之令满口，呼气时慢慢将黑气送至两肾,再入丹田,做 6~12 次。然后,还原至预备式收功。

2. 摩腹吹气法

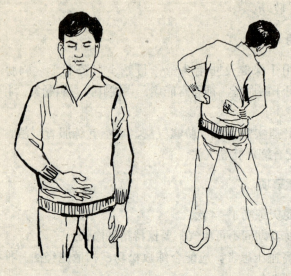

图 43　　　　　　　　图 44

站位或坐位,一手平放于小腹部,慢慢吸气,呼气时口念"吹"字诀,手掌同时轻摩小腹部(见图 43),做 10 息或 20 息。

3. 壮肾导气法

(1) 站位,两手握拳,抵住两侧腰部软肉处,以腰为轴向左转 6 圈(见图 44),再向右转 6 圈。

(2) 搓肾府。站位或坐位,两手在腰部两侧向下推搓 36 次,意存腰部。

(3) 兜肾囊。右手托兜阴囊,左手掌平按于耻骨联合下阴毛处,两手同时一托一兜,做 81 次,然后再换手托兜 81 次。

应用

1. 用于保健或防治腰脊疼痛、耳鸣、耳聋、小便频数、形寒怕冷、阴寒阴湿等症。适用于肾炎、神经官能症、膀胱炎等病。

2. 肾虚者，应练服黑气功，若下焦湿热而致阴湿、阴痒等宜练摩腹吹气功，虚实症均可与壮肾导气法合练。

3. 中老年人，经常练搓肾府、兜肾囊两法有助阳健肾的作用，久久行之必有效。若肾阳虚弱、腰脊痛软、遗精、阳痿者，也宜常练此功。

注意事项

1. 每天早晚各练一次，也可增加至4次。
2. 起居有常，节制房事，青年人治疗遗精、滑精等症，要杜绝手淫的习惯。

3.19 周天自转功

周天自转功，又叫法轮自转或行庭，是以脐为中心，用意念、呼吸，配合默念字句，导引气机循环周转的功法。

功法

1. 预备：坐位或仰卧位。全身放松，自然呼吸，舌抵上腭，意守肚脐部。

2. 以肚脐为中心，吸气时运动腹肌，以意领气。从右腹下侧向上向左旋，默念"白虎隐于东方"；呼气时从左腹上侧，自上向下向右旋转，默念"青龙潜于西位"；如此循环一圈。以脐为中心，顺时针方向，从小圈到大圈，经36圈而至腹之侧。再向反方向旋转，吸气时从左下腹引气向上向右旋转，默念"青龙潜于西位"，呼气时从右上向左下旋转，默念"白虎隐于东方"，逆时钟方向旋转，从大至小36圈，再回至脐部，如此为一次练功。

3. 初练以呼吸及腹肌之力量引动气机旋转，等练熟了，只用意念即可引动内气绕脐轮旋转。练完功再以手掌在腹部顺时针方向转摩 36 次，再逆时针方向转摩 36 次，收功。

应用

1. 本功法可用于中老年康复保健，防病之用。
2. 该功法对消化系统疾病，如胃及十二指肠溃疡、胃炎、肠炎、肝炎等有较好的疗效。如腹胀、腹痛、伤食、便秘、大便不畅等属实症者，可以只向顺时针方向旋转 81 次。如泄泻、少食、四肢乏力等属虚症者，可以只向逆时针方向旋转 81 次。
3. 若与腹部功配合锻炼则效果更佳。

注意事项

1. 用于保健每日练 2~4 次；用于治疗每日 4~6 次。
2. 本功法除所规定的练功时间外，在工作学习之余便可练一会，或疾病的症状加重时即练功，至症状减轻时为止。久而久之对调整身体内之阴阳，有很大的好处。
3. 练功时要轻松舒适，不可闭气，精神不要紧张。
4. 练功前一定排除大小便，不能有一点便意，否则将造成清浊不分之病。
5. 饮食有节，不可过饱，饱则气滞；不可饥饿，饥则气行无力。

3.20　周天功

周天功，又称大、小周天功、内丹术，是健身延年的重要功法，这里只介绍小周天功的练法。

功法

1. 预备：取盘坐式，或平坐式，含胸竖脊，悬顶松肩，两目微闭，舌抵上腭，呼吸调匀，排除杂念。

2. 先采用顺腹式呼吸、练熟之后，再练逆腹式呼吸。呼吸要求调至细、软、绵、长。意守在丹田（脐下3寸），而不死守。腹肌的起伏升降，与呼吸密切配合，活泼自在为原则。

3. 经过一段练功，在丹田部位有一股温热之气逐渐聚集增多，当聚集到相当的程度，就会自然出现一种热气流动的感觉，这时意念跟随着气的流动，从丹田开始顺督脉，从会阴、尾闾端一直上行至头顶，再下至面颊顺任脉下降至胸腹，仍然回到丹田穴，此为一个小周天。

4. 每次练功完毕，都要意守丹田片刻，使气归原，然后搓搓手、搓搓脸，即可收功。

应用

本功法主要用于康复保健，也可以作为一些慢性病患者的治疗疾病的基础功。

注意事项

1. 每天练2~4次，每次10~60分钟，根据锻炼和适应情况，逐渐增加。

2. 练功前要宽解腰带，排除大小便，精神愉快，不可过饱过饥入坐练功。

3. 功夫是自然练出来的，不可过分追求。

3.21 疏肝明目功

疏肝明目功，是疏达肝气，养肝明目的功法。对中、小学学生中的假性近视有较好的治疗效果。有调整视力、放松缓解颈项、背部肌肉和眼肌痉挛，恢复疲劳的作用。

功法

1. 预备: 松静站立, 两脚与肩同宽, 两手自然下垂, 头如顶物, 含胸拔背, 腰膝放松, 两目平视, 呼吸自然。

2. 调视力: 首先两目平视, 由近看至无限远, 凝视一点, 再将视力收回近处, 反复4次, 再平视无限远, 并左右旋视各4次, 自然呼吸。

3. 转颈运目: 两目远视, 转颈, 目光随之旋转, 左右各4次。向后转时吸气, 向前转时呼气 (见图45)。

4. 阔胸松背: 两手屈肘至胸前, 掌心向胸, 两肘后拉, 伸展阔胸, 同时吸气, 然后松背, 同时呼气, 共8次 (见图46)。

5. 按睛明运气: 两拇指按眼内眦内一分处之睛明穴, 意念集中在两眼。吸气时向两眼眶及其后方按压; 呼气时轻挤眼球, 口念"嘘"字 (见图47)。按压以酸胀不痛为度。

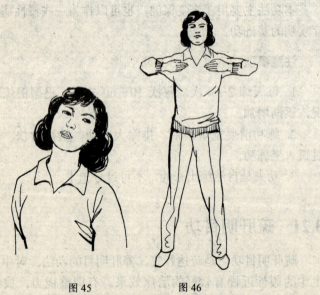

图45　　　　图46

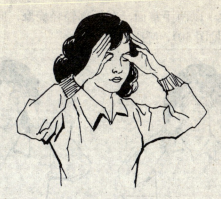

图 47

6. 按上明运气：两手拇指按在眉弓中点眶上缘下的上明穴，意念集中在两眼，吸气时两拇指向眼眶和其后方按压；呼气时轻挤眼球口念"嘘"字。按压时以酸胀不痛为准。

7. 按球后运气：以两中指按眼眶下缘外四分之一与内四分之三交界处的球后穴，食指轻按眉梢后陷处之丝竹孔穴。吸气时中指向眼眶及其后方按压；呼气时轻挤眼球，口念"嘘"字（见图48）。

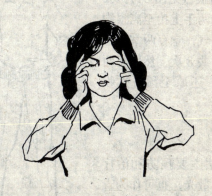

图 48

8. 浴目：以两手四指面轻轻在两目上旋摩，内转8次，外转8次（见图49）。自然呼吸。

9. 浴面：以两手掌面，在面部轻轻旋摩，向前转 8 次，向后转 8 次（见图 50），呼吸自然。

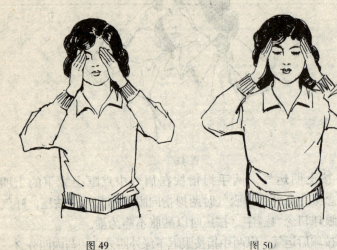

图 49　　　　　　　　图 50

10. 调气：两眼轻闭，屈肘两掌放于腹前，掌心向上，慢慢上提，对准两眼（见图 51）。吸气意存两目，两手上抬至离眼约一拳处，再呼气，意存两掌，下降至小腹部，共 8 次。然后将两手放于两侧，还原至预备式收功。

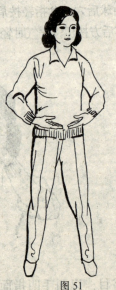

应用

1. 本功法主要预防和治疗青少年近视、散光，也可作为青壮年眼睛保健之用。

2. 练功时要做到排除杂念。

图 51

意念与动作、呼吸密切结合，练功时手掌与眼睛之间似有一种压迫与牵引感、眼皮痒感、眼内温热、清凉等，是练功出现的气感效应现象，不必管它，坚持练下去必有效果。

注意事项

1. 每天早晚各练一次。
2. 避免长时间用眼过度，如需长时间看书学习，劳累时可选练以上功法中几节，以帮助恢复视力。
3. 避免眼睛和目标距离太近，或光线阴暗时看书或卧、立位看书。
4. 经常注意观看远距离的目标。凝视片刻，再慢慢将目光收回。

3.22 养肾回春功

养肾回春功，是中老年养肾健身之上乘功法，有疏通经络、补肾壮阳、延年益寿的作用。

功法

1. 预备：站位，两脚自然分开，与肩同宽，两手自然下垂，头如顶物，脊柱要直，膝松微屈，五趾抓地，舌抵上腭，两目视而不见，排除杂念，松静自然，调匀呼吸，意守丹田，静站3～5分钟（见图52）。

2. 提肛运气：接上势，采用逆腹式呼吸法，吸气时舌抵上腭、缩颈耸肩、收胸、收腹、提肛、同时慢慢提脚

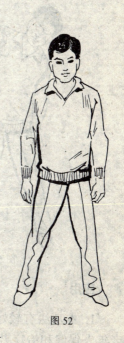

图52

跟,足尖跐地,运气沿督脉上行至顶,呼气时松肛、松腹、全身放松,足跟缓缓落地。运气沿任脉下至丹田,共8次运气上行,意念不可太重,若无气感,意至即可。不可再随意增加次数。高血压患者,意守丹田或涌泉,不运气上行。

3. 八字运肩:接上势,全身放松,自然呼吸,以腰为轴,肩部呈"∞"运转,男先左转,女先右转,左右各8次(见图53),或8的倍数,量自身实际情况而增加。

4. 圆裆振桩:两脚之间比上势略宽,两腿内收肌微用力内收,两膝微微内叩,呈圆裆势(见图54)。呼吸自然,微闭双目,咬肌放松,少腹如忍大便状,以膝微屈微伸,引动躯体,上下振动,牙齿微微撞击,咯咯作响,阴部任其振荡开合,每次5～30分钟,或根据自己身体情况增加时间。

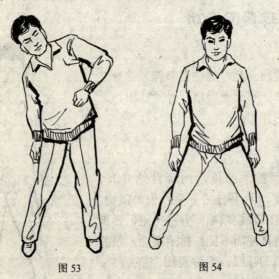

图 53　　　　　图 54

应用

1. 本功法有较好补肾壮阳,强精益气之作用,可以用于中老年人保健和治疗男女更年期综合症、阳痿、早泄、精神萎靡、四肢乏力、发白早衰、记忆力减退等症。

2. 本功法可以配合腰腹导引功。铁裆功等练习。

注意事项

1. 练功时间：每日早晚各练一次，若用于治疗疾病，可适当增加锻炼次数。
2. 生活起居要有规律，节制房事。
3. 练功前要排除大小便，穿松宽的衣服，最好穿大裆裤练功。
4. 注意松静自然，防止邪念丛生。

3.23 采日精月华功

功法

1. 采日精法

(1) 预备：站位，两脚与肩同宽，松静站立，将呼吸调匀，排除杂念，面对太阳方向。

(2) 当太阳从地平线上升起时，微垂帘，但尚可望见柔和微红的日光，以鼻吸气，吸太阳之精光，令满一口（意想），闭息宁神，随呼气慢慢咽下，送至丹田，此为一次。如此 9 咽。

(3) 然后松静自然，静守片刻，再自然活动，即可收功。

2. 采月华法

(1) 预备：夜晚到空气新鲜，空旷之处。松静站立，调匀呼吸，排除杂念，面对月亮方向。

(2) 然后垂帘微见月亮之光，以口鼻吸气，细吸月亮之光华，令满一口（意想），微微闭息凝神；呼气时慢慢咽下，送下丹田，此为一次。如此 6 次。

(3) 最后静守片刻，再自然活动一会，即可收功。

应用

1. 采日精法，适用于阳虚畏寒，四肢不温。脾胃虚弱、精神不振等症。采月华法，适用于阴虚火旺、低热、口渴烦躁、手足心热、腰膝疼痛等症。

2. 用于保健，应根据自己对气的感应情况，灵活掌握练功时间和次数。

注意事项

1. 保健者可于每日初一至初三日寅卯时（5～9时）服日精。采月华则于阴历之十五、十六、十七日服之，每月行三阳、三阴即可。若阴虚或阳虚患者，除以上日期外，其他日期亦可练功。

2. 每逢阴雨大风日不可服气。

3. 患者若经服气，症状基本消失者，可按保健者之法服之。

4. 练功需选择空气新鲜及环境优美之处。

5. 注意精神愉快，避免生气。

3.24 倒阳功

倒阳功，是运用姿势、呼吸、意念，按穴掐诀等法相配合来导引气机的功法。有益肾、培元、练精化气的作用。

功法

1. 夜间阳正兴时，右侧卧位，屈髋、屈膝、向腹部紧收；两拇指掐子纹（见图55），余四指紧握拇指，曲肘放于胸前，闭目垂帘，舌抵

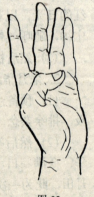

图55

上腭,排除杂念,自然呼吸,意守丹田,静养片刻。

2. 将腰微微向后弓起,用左手中指顶住尾闾穴,右手拇指仍掐子纹握拳。吸气时,提肛、按尾闾、屈脚趾,右手握拳,舌抵上腭,以意引气从龟头沿督脉上至百会。呼气时全身放松,指、趾、肛、舌同时放松,以意引气顺任脉下降至丹田。如此导引气机6息或18息(见图56)。

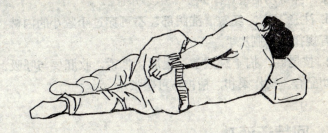

图 56

3. 仰卧位,两上肢自然放于体侧,掐子纹握拳;两腿伸直,吸气时,两脚趾用力卷曲,提肛、收腹、抵舌、握拳,以意引气,用力从龟头向督脉至脑后,上贯顶门;呼气时,腰、腿、手、脚从容放松,松腹松肛,以意引气沿任脉下归元海,反复导气,至阳衰为止。全身放松,意守丹田,收功。

应用

1. 本功法可用于练气保健,练气至气足阳亢之时,以此法练精化气,采药归炉。练功时药至阳兴即行此功,阳衰则止。

2. 防治遗精。遗精多是阴虚阳亢,心肾不交,精不化气,肾不藏精之故。练此功可以交通心肾,练精化气。每于夜间阳兴之时即行功,练至阳衰。或每于夜半子时,免强兴之,再行此功至阳衰,有预防遗精之作用。

3. 本功若与揉腹功、兜肾囊、搓涌泉、铁裆功等配合锻炼则效果更好。

4. 若练功至第二节即达阳衰之效果，就可以收功，不再练第三节。

注意事项

1. 练功要排除邪念，杜绝手淫的毛病。
2. 青年人每月有 2～3 次遗精，若无其他不适，是精满自溢之现象。经练功后会逐渐减少，不必介意。
3. 注意卫生，经常清洗阴部；不可穿过于紧小的内裤。生活要有规律，节制房事。
4. 按尾闾、掐子纹握拳、提肛、抵舌，收肛要与呼吸、意念密切配合。动作柔和，精神不可紧张。

3.25　回精还液功

回精还液功，是升清降浊、回精还液的功法。

功法

1. 预备：每于小便时，调匀呼吸，一手拇指掐子纹握拳，一手持阴器，两脚屈足趾，牙齿叩紧。
2. 当小便撒出一部分时，猛吸一口气，握拳掐子纹，两脚屈趾。同时回缩小便，并从龟头、阴茎向里内收，闭住小便，以意引气内收入命门，复归丹田。然后手足放松再小便，再回缩，一次小便，反复行功 2～3 次。

应用

1. 本功法主要适应于遗精及小便后部出现混浊液体或似精液，小便后尿道不适，睾丸阴茎酸胀、疼痛等症。
2. 膀胱括约肌松弛，小便频数者亦可练此功。

注意事项

1. 练功时间：每于小便时练功。
2. 平时不可忍憋小便、大便。
3. 杜绝手淫的习惯。小便前不要紧张。遗精者可配合练倒阳功。

3.26 涤秽功

涤秽功是祛除大肠邪气的功法。

功法

1. 预备：坐位或卧式，全身放松，舌抵上腭，两目轻闭，呼吸调匀。
2. 意想气从胃口旋入，凭虚而行，将真气运归大肠，驱动大肠热毒垢秽之气，由左绕右，回旋九曲，将秽毒之气旋转送出谷道，然后吸气，微提肛门，使谷道闭住，再自右而左，反方向九曲旋出胃口，共5～10次。
3. 涤秽完要意守丹田片刻，使真气收归原海，以还本原，再揉揉腹，搓搓手、脸，收功即可。

应用

本功法使用于大肠实热症，肠道内有邪毒垢秽之气者，如便秘、腹胀、大肠湿热秽气、腹痛、呕恶、痞满不舒等症。

注意事项

1. 本功法，最好与揉腹壮气功配合。涤秽前先顺时针方向揉腹36次，练功后再按逆时针方向揉36次。
2. 练功时间：每日可练3～4次，症状严重时可以多练些时间。练功时，凡送浊气出谷道外，即随意念吸转，填补真气。

3. 虚症不可练此功法，如阴虚便秘、气虚脱肛、堕胀等。

3.27 铁裆功

铁裆功，是我国古代练下部功夫的重要功法。近代将此功法应用于中老年保健，以及防治阳痿、早泄、遗精，男性不育症等，取得了显著效果。有补肾壮阳、益气养精、强健身体的作用。

功法

1. 推腹：仰卧，全身放松，调匀呼吸，排除杂念（下同），两手相叠（左手在下），自剑突部位向耻骨联合（见图57），推摩36次。两手向下推时慢慢呼气，意念随着手掌的推动，体会手下的感应。有健脾和胃，引导真气达于丹田之作用。

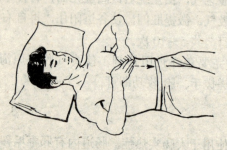

图57

2. 分腹阴阳：仰卧，以两手掌自剑突部位向腹两侧分推36次（见图58）。向下分推时慢慢呼气，注意体会手掌下的感应。有和胃消食，理气健脾的作用。

3. 按揉肚脐：仰卧，两手重叠（左手在下），在脐部左右旋揉各36次（见图59）。自然呼吸，意注掌下感应。有健脾益肾，温阳散寒之作用。若触知腹部有硬块（一般在脐下），是气滞血瘀，结而不散之故，应以食、中、无名三指按住硬块久久按揉，不计其数，并用意向硬块处呼气，使之疏通其经络，消散其积结。

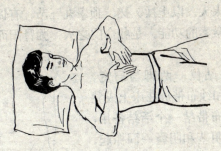

图 58

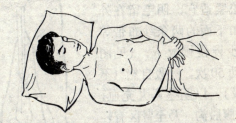

图 59

4. 捻精索：坐位，以两手食、中指与拇指相对，在阴茎根部之两侧捏起精索，左右捻动各 50 次。全身放松，自然呼吸，注意两手捻动精索的感应，以微酸胀，舒适不痛为准。有疏肝鼓舞气机的作用。因手法直接刺激精索中的输精管、血管、神经、淋巴管等组织，故能改善其功能。

5. 揉睾丸：坐位，以右手将阴囊，阴茎一同抓起，虎口朝前，阴茎与睾丸露在虎口外面，将其根部握紧，先以左手掌心按在左侧睾丸上揉 50 次，然后换手，以同样的方法揉右侧 50 次。呼吸自然，将意念集中在揉睾丸那只手的手心里。

6. 搓睾丸：坐位，以两手食、中指面，分别托住同侧睾丸的下面，再以拇指按压其上面，左右搓捻 50 次。

7. 顶睾丸：坐位，以两手食、中指面托住同侧睾丸，再以两指端将睾丸向腹股沟方向顶上去，然后放下来，共 3 次。向上顶时慢慢吸气，放下时慢慢呼气，两腹股沟处有轻微的撑胀感即可，压力不可太大。以上揉、搓、顶睾丸三节，有促进精子的生成和分泌男性激素的功能，是壮命门之火，强肾阳而益精气的重要手法。

8. 挂裆：站位，两脚与肩宽，将备好的沙袋和纱布带放在床上或凳子上，并将纱布带结一个活结备用，然后用一手将阴茎和阴囊一同抓起，再将纱布带的活扣套在阴囊和阴茎的根部扎住，松紧适宜，阴毛留在外面，并使扎扣下面的两条纱布带等长，最后将沙袋慢慢放下，（见图60），前后摆动 50 次，呼吸自然（不可用腹式呼吸），以阴茎睾丸充血，微酸胀，两侧腹股沟，乃至肾区有轻微酸胀和牵引感而不痛为准。本节是对男性生殖器官睾丸、附睾、阴茎、阴囊、输精管、前列腺及阴部神经、血管、淋巴管等组织的综合刺激。可使整个阴部气血充盈，改善其营养，促进其功能。有濡养宗筋，充益精气，壮命门火的作用。

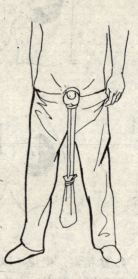

图 60

9. 捶睾丸：站位，两脚与肩同宽，两手握空拳，交替捶打同侧睾丸各 25 次，用力柔和，不可用蛮力捶击，以酸胀不痛为佳。本节能将阴部充盈的气血，引归于肾，滋养肾精。

10. 捶肾：站位，两脚与肩宽，以拳背交替捶击腰部同侧肾区各 50 次（见图61）。动作要柔和深透，呼吸要自然。腰为肾之府，故本节能益肾强腰，并使气血归藏于肝。

11. 通背：站位，两脚与肩同宽，两手握空拳，肩、肘、腕关节放松，以腰的力量带动两手，一手以拳心捶击胸部，一手同时以拳背捶击背部肩胛骨下方，左右各 50 次（见图 62）。本节有通调周身经络，并使气血疏散至周身的作用。

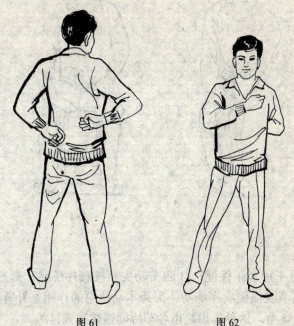

图 61　　　　　　　　图 62

12. 扭膝：两脚并立，以手掌按膝上，左右旋扭各 25 次（见图 63），有通调足三阴三阳经气的作用。

13. 滚棍：坐位，两足穿平底鞋，踏在圆木棍上，前后滚动 50 次（见图 64）。本节按摩涌泉，有导气下行，引火归原之作用。

14. 收功：两手自然放在大腿上面，静坐片刻，再搓搓脸和手，站起来自由活动一下，即可收功。收功之目的是使气血复归于原，精、气、神才不致于散乱。

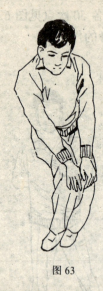 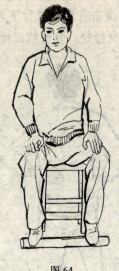

图 63　　　　　　图 64

应用

1. 用于中老年保健，十四节功夫要按顺序练完，最好不要选择练几节或颠倒次序练功，因为本功法总的作用是补肾壮阳，疏通全身气血，这种作用是由各节协同锻炼达到目的。

2. 本功可作治疗一些慢性疾病的辅助功法，如高血压，半身不遂，肝硬化，神经衰弱，慢性胃炎，结肠炎等。

3. 对治疗阳痿有较好的效果，特别是对精神性的阳痿效果更好。第八节挂裆摆动次数，不宜再增加，沙袋重量，可根据自己的承受程度适当增加，当练得阴茎能勃起时，可加练握法，其方法是练完挂裆后，一手握阴茎，龟头露在外面，再努气用力，使气血上达龟头，反复数次。握力和次数逐渐增加，但不可上下滑动或摆动。

4. 练本功治疗早泄、遗精时，患者阴茎易于勃起，或者有欲射精之压迫感时，要用坚强的毅力，排除杂念，并用以下方法进行处理，使其萎缩，欲感消失，再继续练功。方法是：先以两手握空拳，捶击腰部两侧及骶部，兴阳即衰；或兼练捏挣法，是用一手食、中指并拢，放在阴茎包皮系带处，拇指放在冠状缘上，对称用力捏挤，同时一手握住阴囊和睾丸向下拉，数秒钟后，同时放松；再捏拉，至欲感消失为止。

5. 不射精者，可以不练挂裆，而改为双手合搓阴茎，再托兜阴囊睾丸。不育症患者，4至9节加倍锻炼。

注意事项

1. 最好在医生指导下练功，切忌急于求成。先练一百天，在练功过程中禁止性生活。有阴部手术疤痕，输精管结扎，阴部严重静脉曲张，及急性睾丸炎、附睾炎等，不宜练本功。

2. 准备沙袋、纱布带，圆木棍等用具。沙袋为长20厘米，宽17厘米的布袋，装入沙子1.3公斤至2公斤，将口扎紧。纱布带长85～100厘米，宽33～40厘米，将两端缝在一起，使成环形（见图65）。圆木棍长55厘米，直径3.5～5厘米（见图66）。

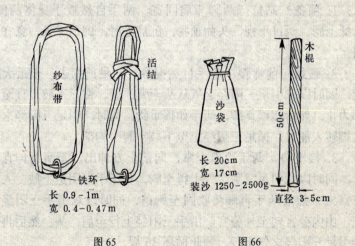

图65　　　　　　　　图66

3. 练功前排除大小便。每天练功 1~2 次。练功以轻松舒适为度。初练腹股沟、睾丸等组织微有胀感，是正常现象，一般 6~7 天消失。如反应严重，可减少练功次数。

4. 精神要愉快，有信心，相信自己的病能够治好，不要过分追求阴茎勃起这一目的，消除性恐惧感，积极练功治疗。肾气强盛，疾病自然痊愈。

5. 练功后睾丸、阴茎、会阴部、或少腹部疼痛，是练功不得法，或次数太多，或挂裆重量增加不适当，造成局部轻度损伤，气血聚而不得消散所致，一般减少练功次数，或暂停练功即可消失。

3.28　升降阴阳导引功

升降阴阳导引功，是导引足三阴三阳经及手三阴三阳经，使阴阳平衡，以祛病延年的功法。

功法

1. 预备：站位，两脚与肩同宽，两手自然放于身体两侧，舌抵上腭，两目平视，头如顶物，沉肩垂肘，调匀呼吸，意守丹田。

2. 缓缓向前弯腰，两手自然握拳，向足前探去，至最大限度，同时以意引足三阳经之气从头至背、腰、臀、下肢，直至足部为止。然后缓缓直腰，两手如握重物。同时，引足三阳经之气入脚转入涌泉，循足三阴经上至下肢、腹、胸部。

3. 接上势，两手由拳变掌，向前上方伸出，至两臂伸直为止，同时以意引手三阴之气上行至胸，再循手三阴达上肢，入内劳宫穴。然后两手再顺势收回至胸前，同时以意引手三阳经之气，由内劳宫转至外劳宫，沿手三阳经上行至肩、头。然后再握拳引足三阳经之气下行，如此循环 36 周。

锻炼中，配合呼吸，引足三阳经之气下行时呼气，引足三阴经之气上行时吸气，引手三阴经之气下行时呼气，引手三阳经之气上行时吸气。意念随经气运行。

应用

1. 本功法能通调十二经之气机，主要用于健身，也可作为一些慢性病治疗期间的辅助功法。
2. 若练此功法后，再配合练十二经之导引功法，效果更好。

注意事项

1. 本功法最好在练通任、督脉导引功后练习，调十四经气。
2. 每天练功1~4次，可于练动功或静功前锻炼，也可单独练或与通任、督导引功配合练。
3. 行功后要自由活动一下。

3.29 通任督导引功

任督二脉乃人身百脉总会之处。此两脉气机通畅，则百脉通畅。本功法是练气通任督两脉的导引功法。

功法

1. 预备：两脚相并站立，两手自然放于体侧，头如顶物，两目平视，调匀呼吸，排除杂念，意守丹田，静站片刻。
2. 通尾闾：微躬身前屈，约100~110度，两手相握，虚拱前出（见图67），两目平视，视而不见，自然呼吸，意领丹田之气会聚于尾闾，然后以腰部力量，使尾闾部位左右摇摆36次。
3. 开双关：接上势，以左手握拳向前伸出，左足同时向左前方迈半步，微成左弓右箭步，右手四指在前，拇指在后叉腰，如勇士开弓之状,然后以意领气从尾闾运至夹脊双关,左右摇动36次。再以同法换右势摇动36次(见图68)。

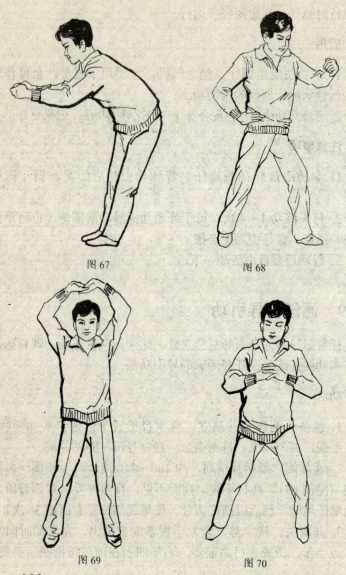

图 67　　　　　　　图 68

图 69　　　　　　　图 70

4. 通玉枕：两脚与肩同宽，两手上举在顶上交叉，掌心向上，足跟微提起，再踏实，反复如舂米之状 81 次，以意领此气自尾闾穴悠悠而起，过夹脊、双关、玉枕，至于泥丸（见图 69）。

5. 气归丹田：接上势，两手握拳，拱手于胸前，与膻中等高。两膝屈曲下蹲（位置高低根据个人的体质情况），如人端坐之状。意领此气从泥丸顺任脉下行至丹田守之（见图 70）。

6. 收功：直立，两手放于身侧，搓搓手，搓搓脸，自由活动一下，即可收功。

应用

1. 本功法能通调任、督两脉之经气，主要用于健身，也可作为一些慢性病治疗期间的辅助功法。

2. 本功法配合周天功、内养功锻炼，有助于练气和打通任、督两脉。特别是练功达气行经络时，再练此功，可助通任、督，防止气功偏差。

注意事项

1. 练功前解除大小便。

2. 练功时间：本功法最好在早晚练习静功或动功前后练功时，效果最好。若无气感，只作意念活动，久而久之，自有气之通调状。

3.30 六段锦

六段锦，又称六段功，是站位锻炼周身经络气血的功夫。

功法

第一段　伸手关洞门

两脚与肩同宽，脚尖内扣，成内八字形，腰腿伸直，两目平视，意守丹田，自然呼吸（见图71）。两手掌向下，慢慢提至胸前两侧，再向胸前方慢慢推出，状如关门；然后腕与十指齐用力向前挣动两臂之筋10次（见图72）。

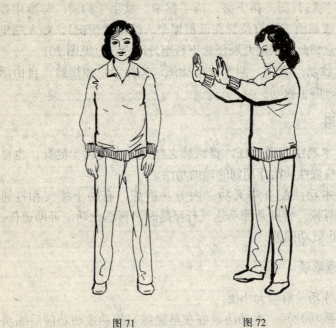

图71　　　　　　　　　图72

第二段　分手耸肩

两臂从前势转为侧平举，当掌心向上，状如担担，两臂齐动后伸耸肩10次（见图73）。

第三段　轻按葫芦

两手由前势收回胸前，然后由上体和两腿自然下垂，掌心向下，手指指向两侧，手掌背屈，用力下按10次（见图74）。

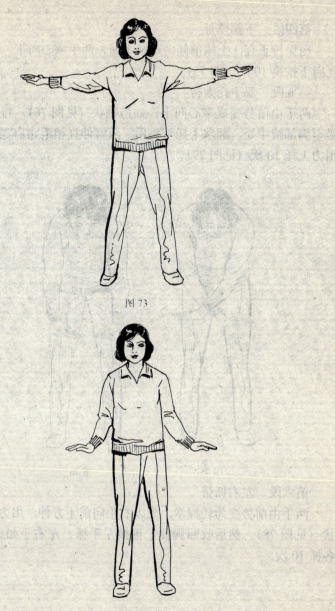

图 73

图 74

第四段　下腰摸丹

腿保持正直，上体前倾，弯腰下屈，两手掌心向下，左右交互向下按摸10次（图75）。

第五段　双手托太行

两手由前势变成掌心向上，如捞物状（见图76），慢慢向上提至胸部膻中处，翻掌上托至头顶，两臂伸直相距如肩宽，然后用力上托10次（见图77）。

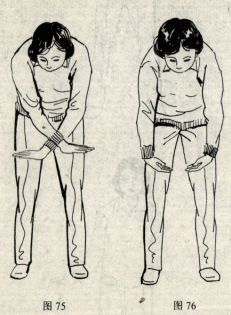

图75　　　　　　图76

第六段　左右抓带

两手由前势变为轻握拳，先以右手向前下方伸，用力如抓物状（见图78）。然后收回胸侧，再换左手抓。左右手如此交替，各抓10次。

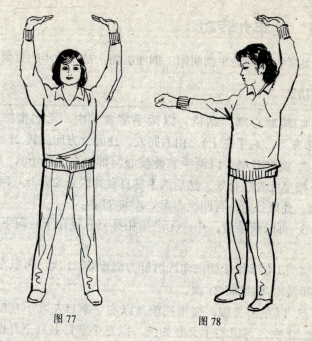

图 77　　　　　图 78

应用

1. 本功是康复保健的重要功法，如练静功后再练本功，则效果更好。

2. 此功有疏通十四经脉之气血，调理三焦，增强腰腿、上肢力量的作用。对腰腿疼痛，四肢关节酸楚，三焦气化衰弱者有较好的较果。

注意事项

1. 每天练2～4次，也可每于练完静功后再练本功。

2. 练功时要穿宽松的衣服，以防影响气脉的运行。

3. 最好用鼻吸鼻呼法，舌抵上腭（也可以吸气时舌抵上腭，呼气时舌放下）。练功完毕，将口中津液下咽至丹田。

3.31 延年九转功

延年九转功是平衡阴阳、调理脏腑、祛疾延年的重要功法。

功法

1. 转摩心窝：站位，以两手掌食、中、无名指按心窝部（左手在下，右手在上），由右向左，逆时针方向旋转21次。

2. 旋推分摩：以两手掌叠按心窝部（左手在下），且旋摩，且下推至耻骨联合处。然后两手掌自耻骨联合处分开，向腹两侧分摩，且摩且走，再回至心窝处，共21次。

3. 再以两手食、中、无名指相叠（左手在下）向下直推21次。

4. 以右手按于脐部向顺时针方向摩脐21次，再以左手按脐向逆时针方向摩脐21次。

5. 以左手叉腰，拇指在前，以右手掌自左乳下直推至腹股沟处21次。再以右手叉腰如前，以左手掌自右乳下直推至腹股沟处21次。

6. 推摩完毕跌坐，两手拇指捏子纹，握拳，扶膝上，将胸自左转前，由右归后摇转21次。再照前法向反方向摇转21次。

应用

1. 本功法有妙合阴阳、调理脏腑，健脾和胃，益气调中的作用。对消化系统之功能紊乱，以及胃及十二指肠溃疡、慢性胃炎、结肠炎、病后身体虚弱、四肢乏力、饮食欠佳等有较好的效果。

2. 适用于中老年人保健康复，可与部位导引功、铁裆功等配合锻炼。

注意事项

1. 每天练2～4次。
2. 练功时最好暴露胸腹部，自然呼吸，注意掌下即可。
3. 动作宜缓和，不可用力推摩。

3.32 易筋经

易筋经是我国古代的一种健身方法。相传本功法的创立和推行，原意是为了锻炼筋肉。顾名思义，"易"是改变的意思，"筋"是肌肉，"经"是方法。就是经过本功法的锻炼，能把萎弱松弛的筋肉改变为强壮结实的筋肉。易筋经重视动作、呼吸、意念的配合锻炼。锻炼起来，气脉流注合度，无迟速痞滞的偏倚现象，是保健强身的上乘功法。

功法

第一式　　韦驮献杵

1. 原文

立身期正直，环拱手当胸，气定神皆敛，心澄貌亦恭。

2. 姿势与要领

（1）左足向左横跨一步，两脚距离与肩宽。两手自然下垂，头端正，两目半开半合，平视前方，舌抵上腭，松肩垂肘，含胸拔背，收腹松胯，膝松微屈，足掌踏实，全身放松，自然呼吸，心境澄清，神意内敛。

（2）两手变阴掌，慢慢地向上抬起与肩平，变阴阳掌向胸前靠拢，两掌心相对，缓缓屈肘，两拇指少商穴轻轻接触，合十当胸，指尖向上。松肩沉肘，用腹式呼吸，气沉丹田，自觉气脉流动时，意念随呼吸，在

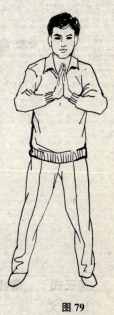

图79

吸气时导引气从指尖而出,进入鼻内,下沉丹田。呼气时,气从丹田上胸,循手三阴经入掌贯指(见图79)。

第二式　　横担降魔杵

1. 原文

足趾柱地,两手平开,心平气静,目瞪口呆。

2. 姿势与要领

(1) 接上式。

(2) 两掌慢慢变阴掌,左右分开,成一字形。同时足跟微微抬起,脚尖点地(功夫深了只用足拇趾点地)。凝神贯注前方,含胸拔背,收腹松胯,舌抵上腭(见图80)。自然呼吸,意念集中于两内掌劳宫穴及足趾部。练纯熟了改用腹式呼吸,在吸气时意念集中于劳宫,呼气时意念集中于足拇趾。

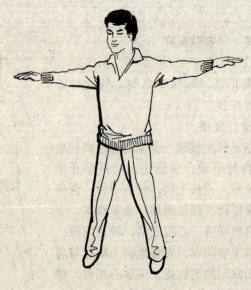

图 80

第三式　　掌托天门

1. 原文

掌托天门目上观，足尖着地立身端，身周腿胁浑如植，咬紧牙关莫放宽。舌下生津将腭抵，鼻中调息将心安，两拳缓缓收回处，用力还将挟重着。

2. 姿势与要领

(1) 接上式。

(2) 两手从左右缓缓向上作弧形上举，将阴掌变成阳掌，掌心向上，手指朝里，直对天门（前发际上2寸）作托天状。同时两足跟提起，微微向外分开，足尖着地，闭合阴跻库（会阴穴）。同时放开膀胱经之会阳穴。牙关咬紧，舌抵上腭，两目用内视法，通过天门，注视手掌之间（见图81）。

(3) 两手握拳，两臂顺原来路线缓缓下降至"横担降魔杵"的架子，开始用鼻吸口呼，后改为鼻吸鼻呼，气沉丹田。呼吸细匀长缓，绵绵不断。吸气时意守丹田，呼气时将意念逐渐转入两掌之间。等气脉运行时，则以意随气。

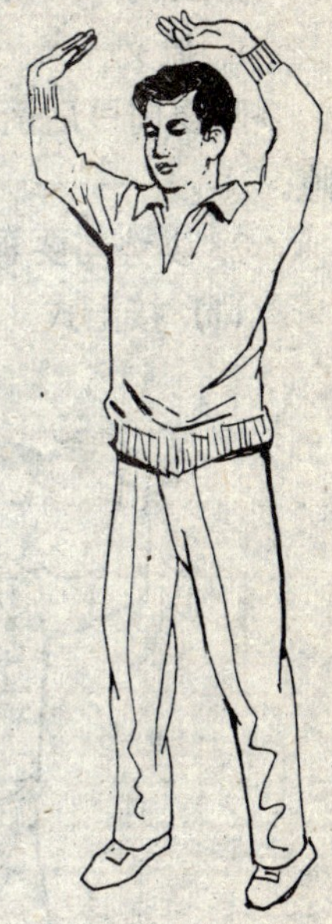

第四式　　摘星换斗

1. 原文

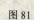

图 81

只手擎天掌覆头，更从掌内注双眸，鼻吸口呼频调息，用力收回左右眸。

2. 姿势与要领

(1) 接上式

(2) 右手向右上方缓缓高举，离额约一拳；同时左手放下，并反手以手背贴于左侧腰眼部。两目注视右手之内劳宫穴（见图82）。

(3) 左手高举，右手放下，手背贴于右侧腰眼处，两目注视左手内劳宫穴，呼吸用鼻吸口呼的方法，把息调匀。意念注视高举之手的劳宫穴，并将内劳宫，两眼，与在腰眼处之手背外劳宫穴连成一条直线，随着呼吸的吐纳，腰眼发生一凸一凹的动作。在呼气时注意内劳宫，吸气时注意下边手的外劳宫。意念内劳宫、眼睛、腰眼随着这种凸凹开合的动作、做微微的运动。

第五式　　倒拽九牛尾

1. 原文

两腿前弓后箭，小腿运气空松，用意存于两膀，擒拿内视双瞳。

2. 姿势与要领

(1) 接上式

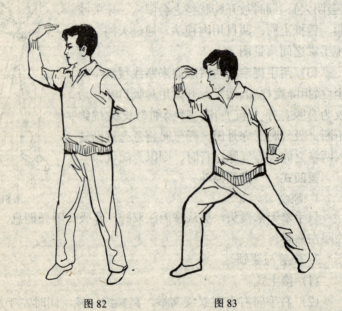

图 82　　　　　图 83

(2) 右手从腰眼离开，微向下垂，顺势变成阴掌向前方抄去，至与肩相平，五指撮拢成"擒拿手"状，腕微屈，指尖朝上向外，劲蓄袖底。同时右腿跨前弯曲，左腿伸直，成前弓后箭步，左手也同时放下，向左后方抄去，右手与额同高，左手与左箭腿成 15 度（见图 83）。

(3) 换左弓右箭步,左手反折抄向左前方,右手收回伸向右后方,动作要领同前。呼吸用鼻吸口呼法,意想两手拉成一条线,似拽牛尾巴之状。吸气时,两眼内视观注后伸之手,向前顺牵,与少腹丹田的气运开合相应地运动着。两腿和腰、背、肩、肘的身段,亦都随着倒拽和前牵的韵味相应地颤动着。如此反复操作3～5次。

第六式　　出爪亮翅

1. 原文

挺身兼怒目,推窗望月来,排山还海汐,随息七徘徊。

2. 姿势与要领

(1) 接上式。借前手向后倒拽之势,前腿后收,两脚并拢。两手收回,掌指翅立笔直,掌心向外,变成"排山掌",放于胸胁部待势。

(2) 两"排山掌"向前缓缓推出。开始前推,轻如推窗,推到肩肘腕平时,五指用力外分,身体直立闭息,两目张开,不可瞬动眨眼,平直地望着前面,集中意念,观看两掌（见图84）。

(3) 再把"排山掌"缓缓向胸胁内收,贴于左右两侧胸胁处。如此反复作7次。用鼻吸口呼法,向前推掌时,配合呼气,推至前面微停息。开始时轻轻用力,前推至极点,则重如排山。收回时吸气。意念集中于两掌中间。

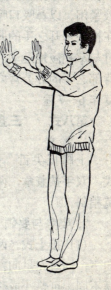

图84

第七式　　九鬼拔马刀

1. 原文

侧首屈肱,抱头拔耳,右腋开阳,左阴闭死,右撼昆仑,左贴胛膂,左右轮回,直身攀举。

2. 姿势与要领

(1) 接上式。

(2) 右手向前提，朝脑后做圆周运动，用掌心贴枕部玉枕关，用食、中、无名三指轻轻压拉左耳的尖端"天城穴"，肩肘相平，右腋张开。左手向左方划，反手以手背贴于脊部两肩胛间，左腋紧闭（见图85）。

(3) 右手放下，反手提起，以手背贴于两肩胛间。同时左手提至脑后，用掌心贴在玉枕关，手指轻轻压拉右耳。左腋张开，右腋紧闭。以鼻吸口呼法，吸气时，意念集中在抱头攀耳之手的肘尖，微微拔牵，头颈同时与掌相应地运动。呼气时意念集中在贴于背部之手的外劳宫穴，气沉入丹田。左右反复作6～7遍。

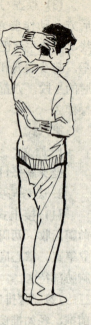

图85

第八式　　三盘落地

1. 原文

上腭抵尖舌，张眸又咬牙，开裆骑马式，双手按兼拿，两掌翻阳起，千斤仿佛加，口呼鼻吸气，蹲足莫稍斜。

2. 姿势与要领

(1) 接上式。两手向左右平伸，与肩相平，成一字形，掌心向下，同时左足向左跨一大步，两脚的距离大约二尺五寸（人高矮不同，可略小或略大些）。

(2) 两膝弯曲慢慢下蹲成骑马裆势，含胸拔背，至大腿与小腿成九十度为标准。在两腿下蹲的同时，两阴掌亦缓缓下按，按压至与膝相平为止（见图86）。动作缓慢，稳稳用力，舌抵上腭，两眼睁大。

(3) 将下按之掌，翻转变成阳掌，如托拿物之状，随两腿的慢慢伸直一起上升，与胸相平为止。如此反复操作 3~5 次。以鼻吸口呼法，姿势下蹲时呼气，上升时吸气，气沉于丹田。意念集中于两手掌，象托拿沉重的东西。

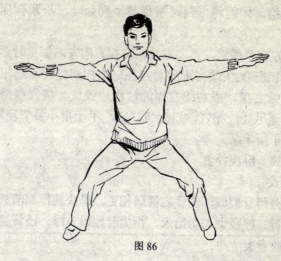

图 86

第九式　　青龙探爪

1. 原文

青龙探爪，左从右出。左掌纠行，跨傍胁部。右爪乘风，云门左露。气周肩背，扭腰转腹。调息微嘘，龙降虎伏。

2. 姿势与要领

（1）接上式。左脚向内收回，至与肩等宽待势。

（2）左手翻掌向下，变成阴掌的"龙探爪"（五个手指的小关节屈曲，掌心空而圆）。用腰部之劲运动，左肘尖领先，向左后方缩去；同时右掌也翻转向下，变

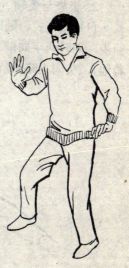

图 87

成阴掌的"龙探爪"。借左掌后伸的姿势，右掌如乘风破浪一般朝左侧面探爪，将左期门穴、云门穴放开，右边的期门穴、云门穴闭着。随着左掌后缩，右掌左探，腰部、腹部相应的扭转，同时要放得很松，才能将"带脉"锻炼得柔韧如丝，松紧合度（见图87）。

（3）左探爪做定，再向右缩、右探。向左右探爪时要同时发出"嘘"音相配合，头颈亦跟随着左探、右探动作转动，用鼻吸口呼法。左缩右探，或右缩左探的过程中吸气，将气缓缓送入丹田。缩探至尽处，呼气，口念"嘘"字，手十指小关节轻轻一抓，意念集中于两手掌。

第十式　卧虎扑食

1. 原文

两足分蹲身似倾，左弓右箭腿相更。昂头胸作探前势，翘尾朝天掉换行。呼吸调匀均出入，指尖着地赖支撑。还将腰背偃低下，顺势收身复立平。

2. 姿势与要领

（1）接上式。随即抬起右腿，向右前方跨进一步，成右弓左箭步，同时两手向前，五指着地，掌心悬空（初练可用整个手掌着地），头向上略抬（见图88）。

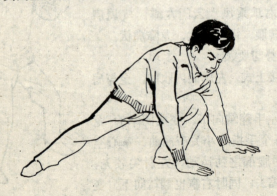

图88

(2) 前足收回,足背放于后足跟上,先做一个俯卧撑,再下俯,臀部慢慢向后收,两目平视,腰部放松,似虎扑食之准备动作(见图89)。

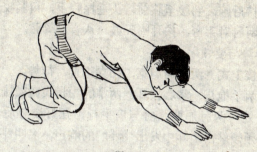

图 89

(3) 头昂起,前胸以低势(约离地4寸),头、腰、臀、四肢呈波浪形向前运动。似向前扑食之状,目视前方,至前臂呈垂直时,胸稍挺(见图90),再收回。如此反复3~5次。最后还原成右弓左箭步。

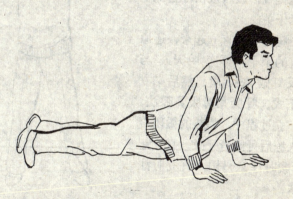

图 90

(4) 作完收回站起,再变左弓右箭,照法做3~5次,还原成弓箭步,后站立成中档(两脚与肩等宽)。

呼吸用鼻吸口呼法,两手扶地,变前弓后箭步,用意调匀呼吸,撑起、前冲吸气,下俯、后缩呼气,意凝注前方,有向前扑捉之意。

第十一式　　打躬击鼓

1. 原文

两掌持后脑，躬腰至膝前，头垂探胯下，口紧咬牙关，舌尖微抵腭，两肘对手弯，按耳鸣天鼓，八音奏管弦。

2. 姿势与要领

（1）接上式。两掌与肩宽，站立正直，待势。

（2）两手抱头，掌心按耳，两掌的中指尖微微接触指头贴在"玉枕关"处。两肘屈曲，肘与肩平行，摆好姿势后，食指击打"玉枕关"频频敲击。耳中发出"隆隆"的响声，名叫"鸣天鼓"（见图91）。

（3）鸣天鼓之后，双手抱头，慢慢俯身，弯腰，将头向两膝的空裆中间弯垂下去，以不能再弯为度，两腿挺直，腰胯放松，舌抵上腭，咬紧牙关。

（4）腿即慢慢直立起来，还原全身笔直的架子，再度"鸣天鼓"与下弯。反复做3～5次。然后站立正直接下式。呼吸用鼻吸鼻呼法。在弯腰直立过程中，慢慢的微闭着呼吸（久练后可闭着呼吸，直立起来）。弯腰时注意丹田，直立时注意两手掌。

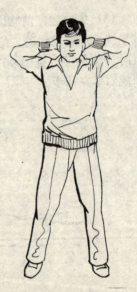

图91

第十二式　　掉尾摇头

1. 原文

膝直膀伸，推手及地，瞪目摇头，宁神一志，直起顿足，伸肱直臂，左右七次，功课完毕,祛病延年，无上三味。

2. 姿势与要领

(1) 接上式。

(2) 将两手从脑后正前方推出去，使两臂伸直，与肩相平。

(3) 将两掌十指交叉扣起，掌心向地，慢慢向胸前收拢，至与胸两拳远时，随即慢慢下推及地，两腿挺直，随即前、左、右各推一下，头亦随之摇摆（见图92）

(4) 再缓缓伸腰，两掌同时上提，双掌松开，向左右各摆动7次。同时，两足各顿地7次，全式用自然呼吸，在推掌及地时，意念集中在两掌心，直立时意念集中于鼻尖。

应用

易筋经是保健强身和发放外气的基础功。青壮年练功有明显的防病健身作用。

注意事项

1. 本功法每天练1～2次。

2. 初练首先要将姿势练熟，然后再进行呼吸，意念和姿势的配合锻炼。

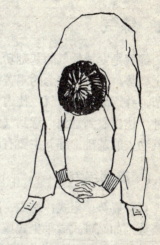

图92

3. 中老年人练此功，不可向上提气，提足跟之动作可以不做，否则易引起血压升高、头痛、头晕等。

4. 本功法是发放外气练气中的动功之一。

5. 每节锻炼的次数，要根据个人的体质和体力情况灵活掌握，逐渐增加，不可操之过急。

4 发 放 外 气

4.1 练气

练气是发放外气的基础功夫。医者首先经过长期静功和动功一定姿势、呼吸、意念的艰苦锻炼,使体内气机的升降开合得到调节,并逐渐积蓄内气,使内气充实,下沉丹田,气脉运行周遍全身,达到心到意到,意到气到,气到力到的目的,就打下发放外气功夫的基础。练气主要有静功、动功与按摩导引功。

4.1.1 静功练气

(1) 姿势:坐式、站式、卧式都可以,从中选择适合于自己的姿势。如站桩式或平坐式或盘坐式,选其一种作为主要练功姿势,其他坐、卧、站式作为辅助姿势,有机会就顺势进行锻炼。要领与方法见第一章。

(2) 呼吸:练气以逆腹式呼吸为主。开始从自然呼吸、顺腹式呼吸练起,等呼吸练顺了以后,就可逐渐过渡到逆腹式呼吸。呼吸锻炼的要求是深、长、细、匀。它是练呼吸功夫的积累,不可勉强为之。

(3) 意念:静功练气的意念,主要采用意守丹田的方法,即"凝神气穴",使丹田之气充实,周天开通。

(4) 练功方法

a. 摆好姿势,全身放松,排除杂念,首先意想自己身体内之浊气,随呼气从全身毛孔、口鼻吐出,共 3 口,再叩齿 36 遍,搅舌咽津 3 口,然后意想天地之清气随咽津而下至丹田,充养全身。

b. 调匀呼吸，意守下丹田，要求自自然然，活活泼泼，不可闭息或者死守，要做到勿忘勿助，顺其自然。

c. 练养相兼，有条件最好培养子时、午时练静功的习惯，其他时间可以养气为主。当然，一次练功中，也要注意练与养相结合。所谓练，就是集中注意力，排除杂念，充分利用有为之呼吸和意念进行练功。养是指用无为之呼吸和意念，以轻松舒适、自然而柔绵的呼吸，注意力集中的静养状态。如在练功中，运用逆腹式呼吸，意守下丹田去练功，已经达到了入静状态，身体轻松，呼吸柔绵匀细，此时可养。只有这样以练养相兼的方法进行练功才能收到好的效果。

d. 气生丹田，周天运转。经过一段时间的锻炼，在练功时丹田气足，便觉有压迫感、温热感或气团移动感等异常而舒适的感觉。日久丹田气感越来越足，在练功静定时，丹田发热，并觉一股暖流从丹田向尾闾骨处冲击（有时会阴穴先跳动，有种周身软绵舒适的感觉），此时要以真气，使其沿督脉向夹脊关、玉枕关循行，至百会，后经任脉，下至丹田。其原则是，气不动我意守之，气将动我意先动。此时用意念配合呼吸使真气在任督两脉循行。吸气使气顺督脉升入上丹田，一呼使气下归丹田为一周。久而久之，练功入定静之时，丹田气升，自不外驰，自然按任督两脉周天循行，此时已不用着力于呼吸的导引，在意念的作用下周天自然转动。

e. 一次功夫练完要认真收功，将意念慢慢移开意守的部位，引气归于下丹田，周身放松，慢慢睁开眼睛，行自我按摩导引之功夫。

f. 自我按摩导引：搓手、浴面、梳发、引行十二经。上肢三阴经从胸搓至手，三阳经从手搓至肩、头侧，下胸腹；下肢三阳经从腰臀搓至足；三阴经从足搓至腹。各搓摩导引10次。然后自由活动一下就可以了。

4.1.2 动功练气

动功练气,是发放外气导引功法的基础功夫。静功是使内部积气、壮气,而动功则外练经络筋骨,使其气脉通畅,运行自如,为练导气功法打下基础。

易筋经:见 3.32 节。

九九阳功

九九阳功是在练易筋经的基础上,采用震桩的姿势,使丹田之气鼓荡,并按一定的姿势、呼吸、意念、使气在周身运动,以增强体质与气的活力,是点射形发气手法的基础功。

(1) 预备

a. 基本裆势

基本裆势是中裆震桩式。

松静站立,两脚与肩同宽,五趾着地,两手自然下垂,头如顶物,两目平视,视而不见,舌抵上腭,沉肩垂肘,前胸微挺,后臀微收,膝放松微屈,精神贯注,自然呼吸。

站定后先如练静功之法,吐浊气3口。然后以膝关节的微动屈伸,引动丹田乃至全身震动,开始震动之幅度大,也不自然,经过一段时间的锻炼后,震动自然,使震动向丹田收拢,然后以丹田为中心震颤,四肢不震动或微震动。震动要自然,震幅要小。以下各式均在此震桩下进行。

b. 柔带脉

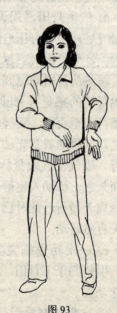

图 93

接前中裆震桩式，作以下功势的锻炼。两手放于带脉右侧处，掌心向带脉，配合逆腹式呼吸，进行手的运行。吸气时左掌在前，右掌在后，推动带脉之气向左侧旋转，意念随手，体会气感，两目微闭；内视带脉。呼气时，右手在前，左手在后，推动带脉之气向右旋转，内视、意念同上，共9息（见图93）。然后用同样动式，引带脉气，吸气向右，呼气向左，转9息。

练功时呼吸、姿势、意念要配合好，腰部要充分放松，以手的气动，带动腰作自然小幅度的旋转。练功中自觉腰软绵如丝束，带脉温热，气行腰周。全身经络气脉活跃，通畅。

c. 三田开合

取中裆震桩式，吸气时两手背劳宫穴相对，慢慢向两侧分开，约与肩同宽。同时收腹提肛，意念、两手与丹田成为一体，感应之气收入丹田，口鼻呼吸浩然之气，亦下沉丹田。共9息（见图94）。

然后两手移至中丹田（膻中）处，以同法在中丹田开合9息。吸气时提气中丹田，呼气时使真气下沉于下丹田。

最后两手移至上丹田（印堂）处，以同法在上丹田开合9息。但吸气时初练内气只提至中丹田，逐渐练习提至上丹田；呼气时气沉下丹田。

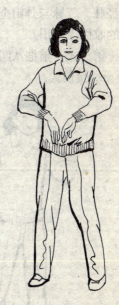

图94

(2) 姿势练法

各姿势练法仍以中裆振桩式进行，但必须振桩与姿势柔为一体，使气运达到姿势之动作上去。

第一式　仙人指路

a. 吸气时收腹、提肛,从下丹田提气至中丹田,两手随之上移屈肘仰掌,置腰之两侧,掌心向上。

b. 呼气时运气于右上肢,四指并拢,拇指伸直,手心内凹,腕关节微背伸上翘,随运气之力肘臂运动内劲立掌向前推出,劲蓄小鱼际处。

c. 吸气时握拳收回胸前,变俯掌下按,左手仰掌提气至中丹田。呼气时以同法将左手推出。左右各9息,收回胸前,提气至中丹田,侧掌待势（见图95）。

按：本势是练少阴、少阳经气脉的架子。呼气运动手臂前推,掌心微凹蓄劲于掌,气达小鱼际、小指处,气贯手少阴,少阳经脉。气脉与丹田全身振动之节奏,源源不断的发出与绵绵不断的收回下丹田。

第二式　前推八匹马

a. 接前式。

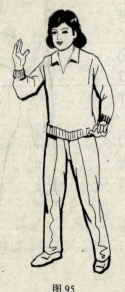
图95

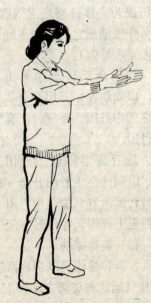
图96

b. 呼气时,运气于肩臂,两掌心劳宫穴相对,拇指伸直,四指并拢，慢慢向前推动，以肩与掌成直线为度，拇指上翘后拉，四指并拢，竖掌下压，气贯四指之指端（见图96）。

c. 吸气时四肢放松，拇指上翘后拉，慢慢屈肘，收回两胁部，再呼气推出，共9息，收回两掌在胸前交叉。

按：本势为练指端活力的架子，运气主要由手太阴、阳明经发出，贯手掌达于指端。练功中指端胀麻，或有热感，是气达指端的效应。

第三式　凤凰展翅

a. 接前式。

b. 呼气时两立掌交叉之手慢慢向左右分开，运气于两臂，十指欲翘，四指并拢，内劳宫有欲突出之势，顺势掌心转向左右两侧，向两侧分推，至肩肘腕平，指仍欲翘，内劳宫欲突（见图97）。

c. 吸气时两掌旋腕屈肘内收，逐渐掌心相对，在胸前之掌交叉。再收回胸两侧，仰掌待势，共9息。

按：本势是练手厥阴及手少阳经之架势。推出时气劲蓄内劳宫，收回时气蓄外劳宫，转而收回丹田。本势久练，气线在掌之周围，其点集中在内外劳宫之间。是运气发气之要势。

第四式　两手托天

a. 接前式。

b. 呼气时两掌缓缓上托至廉泉部，慢慢向外翻掌成两手上托之势托至顶点，指端约距一拳，虎口相对，四指并拢，拇指外分（见图98）。

c. 吸气时旋腕翻掌，指端向上，内劳宫穴对向任脉收回，共9息，两掌仰掌于胸两侧待势。

按：本势是练手三阴经气脉的架子，使气顺手三阴经达于整个手掌面，然后顺手三阳经而下。

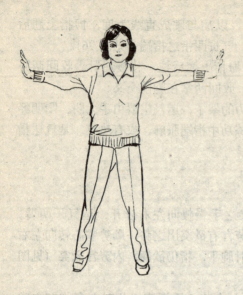
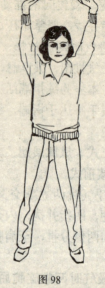

图 97　　　　　图 98

第五式　水中捞月

a. 接前式。

b. 呼气时两手向左右分开，腰前俯下弯，两手像捞物状在两脚间向中点合拢，至指尖距一拳左右，指端蓄劲有托重物状（见图 99）。

c. 吸气时，顺势直腰，抱月至胸前，贯气于丹田，共 9 息。两手俯掌置于胸两侧待势。

按：本势下俯，腰运用柔劲，缓缓而动。两目微闭，视两腿之间有如月之圆者，或一团、一点亮星者，作为月，两手似水中捞物，缓缓集中于此亮处捞起，收入丹田。本势是养丹

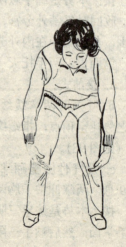

图 99

练肾,通调任督两脉的功夫。

第六势　抱球三揉

a. 接前式。

b. 呼气时出掌右侧,右掌在下成抱球状。吸气时两掌抱球旋扭并向上下微拉,似球充气胀大之状。呼气时微旋扭并按压,似压缩之状,3息。再以同法,右手转上,在中间拉压3息;最后在左侧,左手转上,拉压3息,共9息。两手在左侧抱球待势(见图100)。

按:本势是运气出势的架子。气达两掌间贯足手三阳、手三阴六条经脉,整个手掌似抱球,气脉在两手之间运行。

第七式　运掌合瓦

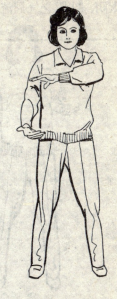

图100

a. 接前式

b. 吸气时左手前伸,右手拉回。呼气时右手向前伸,左手拉回。两手在推拉时导引手三阴之气脉,共9息(见图101)。两手仰掌置于胸两侧待势。

按:本势导引手三阴、三阳经,使气脉达于掌。

第八式　风摆荷叶

a. 接前式。

b. 呼气时两手慢慢向前推,肩、肘、腕相平,左手在上,右手在下交叉,掌心向上。两手阴经与阳经气脉相接。吸气时大鱼际处微下压,向外平分开,顺手太阴经达大鱼际及拇指端。再呼气时小鱼际上翘,气沿手太阳经达小鱼际及小指端,吸气收回胸前共9息或18息。两手仰掌放于胸前待势(见图102)。

· 357 ·

按：本势运动手太阴、手太阳、手少阴、手少阳经之气脉，使太阴、少阳之气周流不息。

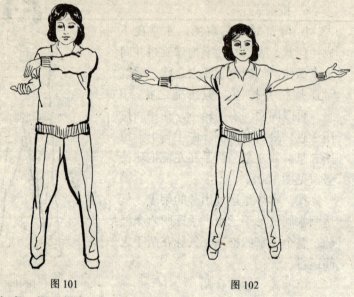

图 101　　　　　　　　图 102

第九式　混元调气

a. 接前式。

b. 呼气时两手仰掌伸出，至肩、肘、腕平（见图 103）。吸气时变侧掌，掌心向外，向两侧划弧，翻掌提气至腋下（见图 104）。掌心向上，指端向胸侧。最后呼气再推出，共 9 息或 18 息。

按：本势调动天地人三气于一体，调合周身之气脉，为收势做准备。

收势：两手相叠，左手在内，右手在上（女相反）放于下丹田处。慢慢停止振动，收气归于丹田。自然呼吸，守丹田片刻。进行搓脸、手及自然活动。

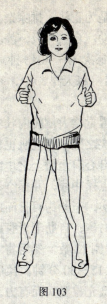 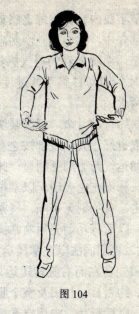

图 103　　　　　　图 104

揉腹壮丹功

揉腹壮丹功，是配合静、动功练气的辅助功法。兼练此功法，五脏坚实，内气壮盛，气积不驰，气力倍增，穴位开合灵敏，不致出偏。特别是练功已成，发功治病之时，不练内壮揉丹之类的功夫，便易致内丹不实，气虚力薄。若此时持续练功,不发气医人之疾，尚能健身延年。若发气医病，因内尚不壮，而气到穴开,卫外之能力不足，故很易受病理之气的干扰而影响自身，造成局部不适，或出现病态，而致周身气机紊乱，使长年练功之成果毁于发功医病。揉腹壮丹功是兼壮内气的辅助功法之一，亦是发功治病者必练之功,若长年坚持必得效益。

（1）仰卧于床上，两腿自然伸直，两手放于体侧，周身、内脏放松，排除杂念，自然呼吸，舌抵上腭。

（2）右手掌（女左手）放于剑突下胃脘处约一掌之大的部位,自右向左旋转揉动（女自左向右,此因男左转顺阳为补，女右转顺阴为补之故）。揉动时不可故意用力而使手僵硬，要自然、柔和，觉掌下腹内有软绵绵之感觉，是为正法。排除杂念，冥心内观，着意守中，意不外驰，勿忘勿助，自然呼吸，静心体会掌下绵绵悠悠，温暖如春的得气感觉。每次 15～30 分钟，逐渐可以增至 1 小时。切勿自感手臂过度劳累，每天早、中、晚 3 次，或早、晚两次。

(3) 约行功月余，气渐凝聚，胃觉增大，腹内壮实，饮食增加，睡眠也好，其中脘部按之有坚实之感，腹直肌也较坚硬或渐隆起，如运气弩力则更明显。此时自心口至脐上之中线，软而有陷，为任脉不充之表现，以掌根重点揉中线，并握空拳自上而下轻轻敲击，久练则无下陷，气亦充实，至此约百日而成。

(4) 以后行功则先用右掌揉腹右侧，自肋下至腹股沟旋转揉运 12 数，再用同法以左掌揉运左腹侧 12 数；然后将右掌放于小腹部丹田处自左而右旋转揉运，约 15～30 分钟。揉后以空拳轻轻拍击。约百日，丹田及整个腹部气充盈坚实而有力。

(5) 以后行功，先用空拳捶击胸之中线及两侧，后施用丹田之揉法，久行胸腹气皆坚实充盈，是为任冲二脉气满。

(6) 此时可运气入督脉，着人协助拍击督脉及膀胱经第一支线与第二支线处，自下而上，自上而下，轻轻捶击，然后以掌根揉之。凡捶后必用掌根搓揉，令其气均润。约百日，督脉之气充满坚实。

(7) 当任督脉充实后，就可自行拍击上肢及下肢，自上而下，重点捶击肌肉丰满处。

以后各部位的捶击手法，亦可使用特制之木棰进行。

当功行约一年，则气周全身，坚实而有力，卫外之机能坚强，穴位闭开灵敏，不致受秽气之干扰。以后每日拿出一定时间揉腹，捶击四肢，以做继续锻炼之用。

4.2 导气

导气，又称运气，是在练气的基础上，再进一步通过导气功法的锻炼，将内气运至发气部位（手式、穴位等），做到意到气到，并能控制、感知内气所到部位的方向、形态、性质，以及气量的大小，为手法发功打下坚实的基础。

4.2.1 合掌震桩导气

(1) 姿势：取中裆震桩式。两脚距离与肩同宽，两肘立掌合十当胸，指尖向上，腕肘相平，头如顶物，含胸拔背，膝胯放松，舌抵上腭，两目轻闭（见图105）。

(2) 导气：自然呼吸，意守丹田，自觉丹田气机发动时（丹田发热，气在运转），呼气时意念随气上督脉，经手三阳经达手掌至指端；吸气时意念随气沿手三阴经返回丹田。当内气循环已通顺，再将意念存于手掌、指端，微微自然呼吸，自觉手掌发热，指端粗胀发麻，微微震动，似有物放出。

(3) 锻炼时间：每日1~2次，每次5~10分钟。

4.2.2 一指禅导气

(1) 姿势：中裆站桩式，左手提起与肩同高，屈腕，食指自然伸直，余指屈曲，拇指与中指相结成环形，右手亦同样姿势，放于右腹侧，两手食指尖相对（见图106）。

(2) 导气：自然呼吸、意守丹田，等丹田气机发动后，随即慢慢呼吸，将气行至右手食指尖，自觉气达指尖时（发热、粗胀感，似有物放出），将气发至左手食指端。感到两食指尖有气牵引时，即用左手的食指点打右手发放过来的气柱，两手有明显的气感；再将气导向左手食指，发气向右手，主动以气柱点打右手食指尖，有明显的气感，再换势以右手在上，左手在下锻炼。

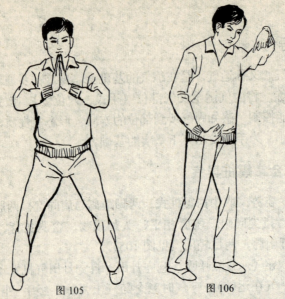

图 105　　　　　图 106

(3) 练功时间：每天 1～2 次，每次 5～30 分钟。

4.2.3　对掌推拉导气

(1) 姿势：中裆站式，两手自然张开，右手自然伸向右前方，左手屈肘在胸前，两掌心相对（左右换手同）（见图 107）。

(2) 导气：自然呼吸，意守丹田，待气机发动后，将气引至左手掌内劳宫穴，发向右手内劳宫，边发边推掌，再将两手掌之气牵引住，顺劲慢慢拉回至原处，两手掌有明显气感（左右换手同）。

(3) 练功时间：每天 1～2 次，每次 5～30 分钟。

4.2.4　三点拉线导气

(1) 姿势：点燃一炷卫生香，放于桌上，或找一物，或在花、树等处。取中裆站式，右手掌自然张开，放在香头前，对准内劳宫，左手成一指禅式，在香头之后方，指尖对准香头，使指尖、香头、内劳宫三点拉成一条直线（见图 108）。

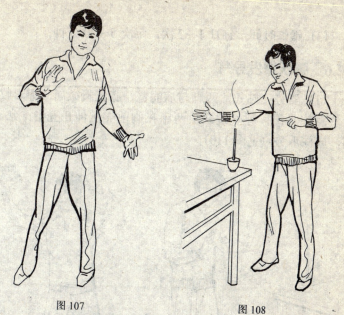

图107　　　　　　　图108

(2) 导气：将食指尖、香头、内劳宫三点拉成一条直线后，自然呼吸，意守丹田，待丹田气机发动后，将气引至左手食指尖，微微呼气，意念转向香头意守住，持续发功，距离先近后远，右手内劳宫有明显的气感。

(3) 锻炼时间：每日1～2次，每次5～30分钟。

4.2.5　三点求圆导气

(1) 姿势：取中裆站式，燃一炷卫生香放于桌上，或放一物，或在花、树旁。两手自然张开，两内劳宫与香头组成一个等边三角形，以三角形的中心为圆心求一个圆，导气时气充满此圆（见图109）。

(2) 导气：用意念将三点求成一个圆后，自然呼吸，意守丹田。待丹田气机发动时，将气引至两手内劳宫穴，微微呼气，发向香头，使三点有互相牵引或撑胀之感，两手似抱一球，再顺气感应，一手牵引，一手顺推，反复练习。

(3) 锻炼时间：每日 1～2 次，每次 5～30 分钟。

4.2.6 腾跃爆发导气

(1) 姿势：站式，两脚与肩同宽，膝慢慢微屈，握拳收气。吸气意注丹田，呼气跳跃，两手在胸前突然伸开五指，掌心向前，成探爪势（见图 110）。

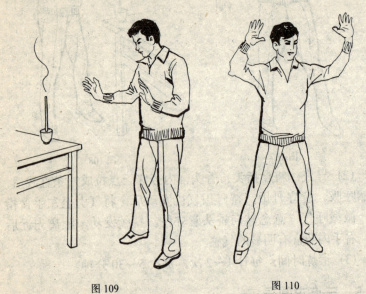

图 109　　　　　图 110

(2) 导气：吸气意注丹田，后提气于胸，收气于掌。呼气时意注掌心，气在内劳宫爆发而出。

(3) 锻炼时间：每日 1～2 次，每次 24 息或 48 息。

4.2.7 点射形导气

(1) 姿势：取平坐式（或站式），坐或站于床边，左手自然放于左膝上，右手伸出以俯掌放于床上，手掌周围接触床面，手心腾起，肘微屈，沉肩垂肘松腕。

(2) 导气：先调匀呼吸，意守丹田，当丹田之气机发动后，运腰微微向逆时针或顺时针方向旋转。吸气时提气至胸，内气震荡，由丹田点滴而上，呼气达掌，由内气的震荡，推动手掌有节律的震动，其频率力量随意念改变。气至手掌，似按球、充气于掌，频频鼓荡，但其点在内劳宫，聚而不散，使气动与手动融合于一体。

本法多取坐式与站式。用中指独立式、探爪式、剑诀式、龙衔式等手式练习震颤点射发放导气。等右手在形体上能震动时，再配合左右手交替之锻炼。本法熟练后可以练习不同频率，不同强弱，不同波峰的气路。

(3) 锻炼时间：每日1~2次，每次30~60分钟。一般3个月可以初步掌握。

4.2.8　螺旋形导气

(1) 姿势：取站、坐、卧各种姿势均可锻炼。以站势为例。取中档站位，右肘屈曲，手掌向前，指端向上，立掌于胸前右侧。

(2) 导气时运动丹田之气，使其逆时针方向运转，等意到气转时，以意念从体内经胸、上肢旋转上行至掌，使丹田与手掌同步旋转。在丹田以脐为中心，在手掌以内劳宫为中心。初练速度宜缓，逐渐加快，要顺其自然，不可强求。本法亦可伸出剑指，或中指以同步锻炼。练时可以从大圈转至小圈，或从小圈转至大圈等不同形式的运动法。

(3) 锻炼时间：本法需充分利用站、卧、坐各种不同姿势，时常锻炼，方可掌握，不是一日之功。

4.2.9　冷热导气

冷热导气的锻炼主要适应于"寒者热之，热者寒之"的治疗原则。

热导气是摆下一定姿势之后，先调匀呼吸，意守丹田，意想丹田之气似火热的太阳，烧遍全身，后将此意念转移至手掌，在手掌中燃烧发热，或在指尖燃烧发热，或在一定的手式中燃烧发热。

冷导气是调匀呼吸，意守丹田，然后下至涌泉。吸足跟地气从下上行达胸至掌，意想手中冷似冰，守之。此法不可意想周身冷似冰，或引向其它部位，否则影响气机的协调。

本功法可在练震桩等导气功纯熟之后，与其他导气功结合锻炼。

以上八节功法，每次选 2~3 势锻炼。练毕静站片刻，将气引归丹田，再搓手、脸。微微活动一会儿，就可收功。

4.3 发气

发气，又叫"发功"、"发放外气"，古称"布气"。是经过练气、导气功法的锻炼，将自身的内气运至指掌，或其他发气的手式，再运用发功手法，使气发放到受气者经络、穴位上的方法。

4.3.1 发气手式

(1) 一指禅式：食指伸直，中指、无名指、小指自然屈曲，拇指屈曲轻压在中指背侧，运气于食指端，接触或离开治疗部位发气（见图 111）。

(2) 平掌式：五指自然伸直，运气于手掌，以内劳宫为中心，接触或离开治疗部位发气（见图 112）。

(3) 探爪式：五指自然张开，指间关节屈曲呈探爪势，运气于指尖，接触或离开治疗部位发气（见图 113）。

(4) 剑诀式：食、中指伸直并拢，无名指、小指自然屈曲，拇指轻压无名指及小指甲部。运气于食、中指端，接触或离开治疗部位发气（见图 114）。

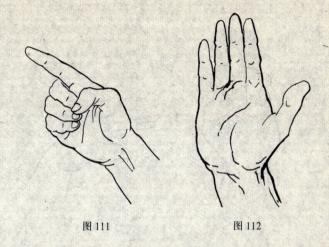

图 111　　　　　　图 112

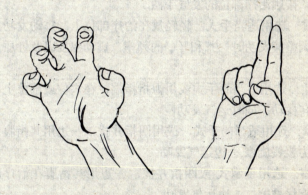

图 113　　　　　　图 114

(5) 中指独立式：中指伸直，余指自然屈曲，运气于中指端，接触或离开治疗部位发气（见图 115）。

(6) 龙衔式：拇指与其余四指伸直相对，运气于拇指与其余指之间发气（见图 116）。

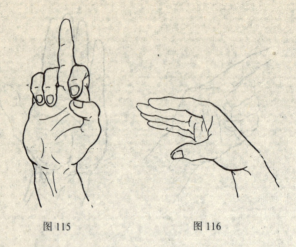

图 115　　　　　图 116

4.3.2　发气手法

(1) 接触治疗部位的发气手法

a 震：选用适当手式，轻轻放在治疗部位上，震动发功。需用意念调整其发功时"力"和"气"的频率、震动幅度以及性质和量的大小。

b 揉：选用适当的手式或用拇指指端，在穴位或部位上一边用力旋转揉动，同时运气发功。

c 摩：选用适当的手式，或用四指并拢，一边用其指腹在穴位上用力慢慢旋摩，一边运气发功。

d 擦：选用平掌式，或四指并拢，一边用其指腹在治疗部位上慢慢直线推擦，一边运气发功。

e 抑：选用适当的手式，放在治疗部位上，垂直施加压力，并运气发功。

(2) 离开治疗部位的发气手法

a 推：选用适当手式，离开治疗部位约 15～100 厘米。用两点或三点拉线、三点求圆等导气法慢慢导气。当有气感时，用内劲轻推，发气于治疗部位或穴位上。

b拉：选用适当手式，离开治疗部位，用两点或三点拉线、三点求圆等导气法，慢慢导气于治疗部位或穴位上。当有气感时，用内劲轻拉，发气于治疗部位上。

c旋：选用适当的手式，离开治疗部位，用螺旋导气法，慢慢导气。当有气感时，手式慢慢旋扭，或左、或右使气旋转导入，发气于治疗部位或穴位上。或用三点求圆导气法，慢慢导气。当有气感时，用内劲一手轻拉，一手轻推，顺圆周运转，发气于治疗部位上。

d颤：选用适当的手式，离开治疗部位，用点射导气法，慢慢导气。当有气感时，手式微微震颤，用点射法发气于治疗部位或穴位上。

e引：选用适当手式，离开治疗部位，慢慢导气。当有气感时，发气于治疗部位上，并根据病情顺经或逆经、或左、或右、或上、或下的导引经气运行。

f定：选用适当手式，离开治疗部位，慢慢导气。当有气感时，采用一种或几种发气方法定点发气于治疗部位上。

(3) 辅助手法

a点：用一指或拇、食、中三指捏拢轻轻点打经络穴位。

b拍：用五指自然伸直，成虚掌拍打治疗部位，或经络穴位。

c击：手握空拳，用手背或其他部位打击治疗部位，或经络、穴位。

d按：用拇指指端或手掌按压治疗部位或经络、穴位。

e抚：用一手或双手掌面，在经络、穴位或治疗部位上推抚。

f拨：用指端在穴位上拨动。

g搓：用双手掌面，或拇指与食指、中指面挟住一定部位，对称用力，轻轻搓揉。

h 摇：用手摇动或扳动肢体关节。

i 搈：以手背近小指处，附着于一定治疗部位上，使腕关节作屈伸外转的连续活动。

4.3.3 发气中的气形

据临床发气体会，在发功治病过程中，紧密配合不同的气形进行发气，是掌握发功治病的关键之一。发功中气的基本形有线、点、旋三种。掌握这三种气形，就可临床随病随气变应，或选用一形，或选用两形之组合，或变化出一些特殊气形。在运用这三种基本形发功时，还可配合气质、冷热等导气方法发气，成为组合式。

(1) 线形：其锻炼方法是以两点、三点拉线及其他一些类似的导气方法为基本功，一般用推、拉、定、引等手法发气。发功较平和，有较明显的压迫感、牵引感、温热感、凉感，是一般导引经气，补其不足，泻其有余的基本形。此气形发功手法一般要稳而缓，呼吸深而自然，或借助于深缓的呼吸发功。

(2) 点形：是常用的一种发气气形，以震桩及点射导气法为基本功。可用各种手法发气。以本气形发功，对经络穴位之气、丹田之气等气机的激发尤为显著，是调动、激发气机的主要气形。

以此气发功多以平坐或中裆站式，用自然缓慢的呼吸，以腰为轴，腹为泵，使自身气机震颤，并导引至发功手式，发功到治疗部位上。其气似滚珠，一粒接一粒地发出，意念随之震颤，并给予一定方向和部位的诱导。

本形发气绝不可并气，或利用肌肉之强力震颤推动手法的震动，否则易造成气滞，而出现胸闷、胁痛、臂似折、肉似裂之弊病，应特别注意。

要掌握好此发功气形，应当将震法练顺，使气自然而发。一般要按练气、导气和震颤手法的顺序锻炼，持之以恒，3个月可望能基本掌握，但尚不能流利地运用于临床，可见此法掌握之难。

(3) 螺旋形：本气形是以螺旋导气手法，导引内气以螺旋形式发放。本形发气以气感深透为其特点，对气机有一种特殊的调节作用。

本气形之发放以自然呼吸，螺旋形意念诱导，其旋波先从丹田起，一环扣一环地走向发功手法，自己能感觉出发功手法处之旋转气流。

本气形除以上发功的锻炼外，当经常练习丹田运转，丹田与手式的同步运转法。要形成一个牢固的螺旋气路。丹田转则手式处即出现气转，可以随意念而转移，得心应手，方能应用于临床。

4.3.4 气感

气感是发气治病中医者和患者各自对气的感应而出现的一种感觉效应。医生可以根据自己的气感与患者的气感来判断疾病和调整手法治疗疾病。

(1) 真气的气感：真气信息多为微微之热、凉、麻、压迫、牵引和气的运行等感觉。多能感知其方向、疏密、性质、大小等。

(2) 秽气的气感：秽气信息的气感又称"病理信息"。此气是一种信息，与现代医学所说之传染病因素不同。可归纳以下几种：

a 寒凉感：此气感特别寒凉，甚或当感知到此气感后从指端迅速发冷，末端血管迅速收缩，指端发冷，并向上传导，或出现战栗、毛孔收缩等。有一种特殊的冷感和不适感。

b 燥热感：此气信息反应到医者手上或身上，有一种燥热的感觉，并有烦意，似火烤。

c 酸麻感：接受到此种气感后，局部麻木不适。

d 秽气感：当医者与患者相对而立，或对坐，或向其发气时，可感知到此种秽气，给人一种特别污浊难以形容的感觉。

e 其他：古有病喜气、忧气等五气，六淫之邪气之说。如有时感受到喜之邪气等也能有所反应，这就要凭医者细心去体会。

4.3.5 气效应

当医者向病人发气治病时，大多数患者会产生一些气效应，主要有以下几点：

(1) 气感效应现象：当医者发气时，有些病人可立即或逐渐在局部产生类似或练功触动样的气感，有冷、热、压迫、牵引、虫爬、麻、重、轻、浮、沉等感觉。这是气行经络和作用于治疗部位而达到病灶的一种气感效应。其中冷、麻、热、压迫、牵引是常见者。

(2) 动态效应现象：当医者发气时，患者可立即或逐渐产生肢体某一部分或整体出现不自主的动态现象。有的是微微的肌肉震颤，有的是肢体大幅度的运动。这是一种外气激发，诱导自发动功的现象。

(3) 光电效应现象：有些患者接受外气后，可出现光电现象。有的表现为肢体触电样感觉，有的微闭其眼，可看见不同形态的光图，多数为圆形，或呈片光形，或闪电样图形。

(4) 声效应现象：有的患者接受到外气后，可听到声响，如"喇喇"、"隆隆"、"吱吱"的声音。

(5) 气味效应：有的患者接受到外气后，可嗅到一种特殊的气味，其反应也不一样，如呈檀香或各种花香等。

(6) 气晕厥现象：有少数患者当接受发气治疗后，或在旁候诊接受到外气后，就出现大汗淋漓，心率加快，出现类似晕针样昏厥现象。有的病人虽无明显气感和动象，也会出现如上之晕厥现象。有的病人经外气激发，出现晕厥后，病机就会有明显的好转。当患者出现气晕厥时，立即仰卧，再用手法轻点百会、命门、肩井、印堂、拿肩井。然后顺任督两脉导引，引气归原，自可恢复。

以上是常见到的气效应现象，其中以"气感"现象最为常见，而"动态现象"则为少数，其他亦少见。

气效应现象，是患者接受外气后，感觉、运动等器官出现的一种特殊现象。它决定患者某感触器官和经络感知的敏感程度，而不能简单地用来测量"气"达病所所产生的治疗效果，有的患者虽无明显的气效应现象，但经几次治疗后疾病恢复很快，同时慢慢也有了气感；而有些患者，气效应现象很强烈，但治疗效果则不甚明显。当然这是个相当复杂问题，有待今后进一步研究。

4.3.6 收功

(1) 给病人收功。发气给病人，就象病人在做功一样，治疗完毕，要根据情况，用点、拍、叩、搓、摇等手法，给予放松、调和等处理，以引气归原。

(2) 医者收功。医生发气完毕，要将气慢慢收归丹田，手式要离开发功部位。适当调整一下自己的意念、呼吸、姿势，使全身放松，真气归原。若被病理秽气干扰，还要先排放秽气，然后再进行调整。

5 治　疗

5.1 气功偏差

气功偏差是指练功过程中出现不良反应，构成痛苦，自己不能控制和消除，而有损于身心健康者。出现偏差的原因大致有以下几种：

1. 没有老师指导，或由既没有练功经验，又不懂医理的人教授功法，练功不得法，或盲目学练某种功法。

2. 不能辨证施功，如体质和病情不宜练内气运行的人而勉强去练。

3. 急于求成，盲目追求练功效应，或精神脆弱，疑心过重，不能正确对待练功过程中的触动和气效应，而形成思想负担，久而久之而成偏。

4. 不能正确掌握和运用练功中的三调原则和方法，或不按功法要求练，选择功法见异思迁，朝秦暮楚，无目的地更换功法，造成功法混乱，思想矛盾。

5. 练功中受惊吓，或思想受到其他刺激而勉强练功。

6. 在练功中盲目地导引内气运行，或内气外放，违犯了自然规律。

7. 练功中出现正常的触动现象，自己疑神疑鬼，或找发放外气者胡乱导引治疗，致使内气激发，气流不止。

5.1.1 气血逆乱

症状：在练功中或练功后出现气脉乱窜，不能自控，引起头晕、目眩、惊恐、胸闷、气短、肢体摇动、震颤，或气在某经某处流动不止，异常不适。患者一般能说出气血窜动的位置和方向。

治疗：

1. 练功自疗

首先停止所练功法，消除紧张和恐惧心理，把意念转移到有益的活动上，再于有症状表现的部位上做自我拍打功，并按手、足三阴、三阳经的循行路线和方向，进行自我按摩导引。症状严重者，要请有经验的气功医师诊治。

2. 外气疗法

(1) 按气机逆乱之部位、经络，选取穴位。用平掌式或剑诀式，以推拉颤等手法，激发该经及相应之经的气机。

(2) 然后以推导手法顺经或按部位导引，调整阴阳，引气归于某经、某脏，或引气归于丹田。

5.1.2 气滞血瘀

症状：在练功中或练功后，由于气机不利，引起身体某一部位气滞血瘀，而出现疼痛、沉重、酸胀、压迫等感觉，不能自行消失，或越来越重。

治疗：

1. 练功自疗

(1) 先停止所练功法。

(2) 泰山压顶。出现头顶压迫感，疼痛难忍者，患者可以自行按摩百会、风府、天门、坎宫、太阳，再顺督脉及任脉循行方向拍打、推摩。再意守涌泉、大敦穴，配合练头面部功。

(3) 出现前额凝贴，紧张者，先开天门、推坎宫、运太阳，并自行从督脉百会穴向下顺任脉拍打至丹田，反复数次。再向下推摩数次，配合练头面功及颈项功。

(4) 大椎胀痛者，推大椎、脊中，并顺督脉向下拍打，反复数次。其他部位的气滞血瘀现象，亦宗上法进行处理，不可乱服发散药，或外气导引，或针刺导气。

2. 外气疗法

(1) 先在气滞血瘀之部位，按邻近和循经选穴法选出穴位点揉之，并顺经推摩。

(2) 用平掌式，以推拉颤手法发气，以激发经气。然后按经脉循行路线顺经导引，导引气机，疏通经络。

5.1.3 真气走失

症状：在练功中或练功后，患者自觉有气从前阴后阴或某些穴位不停地向体外漏气，不能自控。相继出现消瘦，四肢乏力，面色灰暗，心慌意乱，精力不能集中，记忆力减退、自汗、盗汗、遗精、失眠、懒言少动等症。

治疗：

1. 练功自疗

(1) 首先停止练运气功法。可练习提肛、叩齿、咽津等功法。按经脉的循行方向，拍打任督两脉以及十二经脉，使全身气脉通畅。

(2) 服用以下中药，以引气归原：熟地 30 克　山萸肉 30 克　人参 9 克　磁石 30 克　牛膝 18 克　肉桂 6 克　生龙骨 30 克　生牡蛎 30 克　朱砂 1 克（冲服），共服 5～10 付。

2. 外气疗法

(1) 首先点揉肾俞、命门、丹田、关元诸穴。

(2) 用平掌式、以推定手法向命门发气；再用推导手法引导经气归原。前后阴、会阴穴漏气，以壮丹田，导气上行，归于中丹田为主。周身毛孔漏气，以闭穴导气，使气归于膀胱经、肺经为主。鼻窍漏气，以疏通肺经及任脉为主。

5.1.4 神昏颠倒

症状：在练功中出现神昏颠倒现象，称为"入魔"，是将在练功中或在练功后出现的幻景，信以为真，而致神昏错乱，性情孤僻、退缩、呆滞少动，情志淡漠，精神恍惚。或因失去生活的信心而轻生，或幻听、幻视、幻觉，缠绕不断等，类似于精神病患者的现象。在《钟吕传道集》中归纳为十魔：六贼魔、畜魔、贵魔、六情魔、恩爱魔、患难魔、圣贤魔、刀兵魔、女乐魔、女色魔等。

治疗：

1. 练功自疗

(1) 停止所练功。对幻景不予理睬，视而不见，听而不闻，任其自生自灭。严重者请医生做综合治疗，方可收到较好的效果。

(2) 可服百合地黄汤加味：百合 30 克　生地黄 30 克　生牡蛎 30 克　磁石 30 克　牛膝 15 克　远志 12 克　炒枣仁 9 克　朱砂 1 克（冲服）。水煎服。

2. 外气疗法

(1) 按灵龟八法按时开穴法，打开奇经八脉之穴。

(2) 按揉百会、大椎、灵台、肺俞；再用平掌式或剑诀式，以推拉颤引手法发气，并顺经导引之。

(3) 掐百会、印堂、山根、人中、听宫、颊车、曲池、合谷、委中、承山。

(4) 用中指独立式，以震颤手法在鸠尾穴、中脘穴发气 18 息，并顺任脉导引使气归丹田。

5.1.5 练功中暂时反应的处理

由于初练功,对功法的要领掌握不正确,可以出现一些常见的反应,不可作为偏差对待,适当地处理一下即可。现分别介绍于下:

头胀头痛:一般是初练功者不习惯练功方法,情绪紧张、面部肌肉不能放松,或用意念太重所致。处理的方法是,在练功中时刻注意精神及头部肌肉的放松。配合练习头部导引功。也可练放松功、嘘字功。

胸闷:一般是由于呼吸不得法,屏气拉长呼吸所引起的,可以练摩胸呵气法,摩胸呬气法及胸部导引功,或意守足三里,即可消除。

腹胀、腹肌酸痛:一般是初练腹式呼吸,时间过长,或用力过大所引起的。练功中注意腹肌的运动逐渐加大,减少练功时间,再配合练腹部导引功,即可消失。

四肢发冷:多数是由于练功者,阴气盛、阳气衰微,或由于练功的时间、方位、呼吸不对而引起。若练功方法准确,可以不必管它,阳气渐复即可好转。由练功方法所致者,则要采用正确的练功方法,可以配合练采日精功。

5.2 昏厥

昏厥又称晕厥,是一种急速而短暂的意识丧失。主要是由于暂时性脑缺血、缺氧所致。每因情绪过于激动、惊恐、剧烈疼痛、站立过久或骤然起立等而诱发。祖国医学认为属于气机逆乱或气虚下陷,清阳不升所致。

症状:体质素弱,发病时通常先是头昏、眼花、气短汗出,继则昏倒,不省人事,面色苍白,四肢厥冷,血压下降,脉细数,瞳孔缩小等。也可因针刺、推拿手法强烈,或接受外气治疗而导致晕厥者。

治疗：

1. 练功自疗

当出现昏厥先兆时，可用以下自我练功的方法进行自我调整治疗：

(1) 当出现昏厥先兆时，立即仰卧，头略放低些，松解领扣，全身放松，深吸一口气，以意领气送入丹田。

(2) 自己以右手或左手拇指甲掐人中、内关、合谷等穴。

(3) 两手放于身体两侧，自然呼吸，舌抵上腭。以部位放松法，先头部，然后颈项、上肢、胸腹、背腰、下肢逐次放松，练3遍，再静卧片刻即可。

2. 外气疗法

(1) 患者仰卧，全身放松，先掐揉百会、人中、内关、合谷、太冲诸穴，以升阳益气，醒神开窍。

(2) 用平掌式，以推拉手法发气于下丹田、中丹田、上丹田，使气机活跃；再用平掌式推引手法，自百会向前，顺任脉导引气机至下丹田。然后疏通至两下肢，直至两脚，反复3~7次。

(3) 用推抚手法，将两上肢、两下肢顺手三阳经及足三阳经自上向下推抚3遍，以调理气机，疏通气血。

5.3 感冒

感冒或简称"上感"，是由病毒或细菌感染引起的呼吸道炎症。每因气候变化，抗病机能减弱时发病。祖国医学认为感受风寒、风热或时行疠气所致。

症状：感受风寒者，头痛、鼻塞、流清涕、喷嚏、怕冷、无汗、咳嗽痰稀、骨节酸楚、苔薄白、脉浮紧。如属风热者，头痛发热或汗出，咽喉干痛，鼻流黄涕，咳痰黄稠，苔薄而微黄，脉浮数。

治疗

1. 练功自疗

(1) 坐位，或卧位。以拇指按揉印堂、太阳、曲池、合谷诸穴。

(2) 再练头面功、鼻齿功及颈项功之疏导风池法及推导天柱法。

(3) 最后练上肢功及下肢功之通导手三阴、手三阳经及通导足三阴、足三阳经法。

2. 外气疗法

(1) 患者坐位先按揉印堂、坎宫、曲池、合谷以开通穴位，疏通气机。用平掌式，以推拉手法发气于印堂、太阳，并用拉导法、顺任脉、及足阳明胃经向下导气，直至两足，3~7次，使风寒及风热之邪气，顺经下导，自足而出。

(2) 再按揉风府、大椎、风门、肺俞诸穴。然后用平掌式以推拉手法向大椎、风门、肺俞发气，并用拉导法顺足太阳膀胱经自上向下导气，至气机平衡为止。

(3) 最后按揉风池、大椎、风门、曲池、合谷及两上肢结束。

5.4 胃脘痛

本病以胃脘部疼痛为主症。祖国医学认为肝气犯胃、脾胃虚寒、气滞血瘀等，均可导致胃脘作痛。其疼痛发作常与饮食不节、气候变化以及精神因素有密切的关系。与现代医学中慢性胃炎、胃及十二指肠溃疡病相类似。

症状：肝气犯胃者，胃脘疼痛而胀满，呕逆吞酸，情绪激动时更甚，脉弦苔薄白。如属脾胃虚寒者，痛多喜按，得温则减，食少嘈杂，呕吐清水，二便清利，形寒畏冷，苔薄白，脉迟。如气滞血瘀者，其痛拒按而有定处，或有积块，或大便黑色，舌质红，脉弦涩。

治疗：
1. 练功自疗
(1) 选练放松功、内养功。
(2) 肝气犯胃，气滞血瘀者，练理脾功之摩脘呼气法及疏导脾胃法。属脾胃虚寒者宜练理脾功之服黄气法及疏导脾胃法。
(3) 配合练胸胁功及腹部功。
2. 外气疗法
(1) 病人仰卧，全身放松，排除杂念，调匀呼吸。然后呼气时以意引气导向胃脘部疼痛处。
(2) 医者以右手揉阑门、左手中指按鸠尾穴，以调法放通阑门穴。
(3) 医者用平掌式，以震颤法在胃脘部发气14息；再用中指独立式，以震法在中脘、气海发气14息；然后分腹阴阳，推腹，摩腹，揉腹。
(4) 用平掌式，以推拉颤手法离开中脘穴发气14息。再用推引手法顺任脉向丹田导引经气，或顺胃经向下导引气机，达平衡为止。
(5) 患者俯卧揉脾俞、胃俞、肝俞及膀胱经督脉。并在脾、胃俞震颤发功14息。并用平掌式，以拉引手法，自上而下顺足太阳膀胱经导引气机。

5.5 阑尾炎

本病多为阑尾腔梗阻和细菌感染所致。祖国医学称为"肠痈"，认为由于饮食不节，寒温失调或饱食后暴急行走等，导致食滞中阻，肠胃功能失调，或湿热积滞于肠道，气血凝阻而发为"痈"。

症状：腹痛开始多在上腹或脐周围，数小时后移至右下腹（这种转移性腹痛为本病之特点），呈持续性钝痛阵发性加剧。可伴有恶心、呕吐、便秘、腹泻，右下腹阑尾点（在右髂前上嵴与脐连线的外 1/3 与中 1/3 交界处）局限性压痛及反跳痛。体温在 37.5℃ 左右，随着病情发展可逐渐升高。如体温较高，腹痛骤然停止，可能是阑尾穿孔，要及时转外科处理。

治疗：

1. 练功自疗

(1) 患者仰卧位，练放松功，以放松腹部及内脏为主。

(2) 练周天自转功，以意引气，使腹部气机随意念自右向左逆时针方向旋转 18 息。

(3) 练腹部功，手法轻柔。

2. 外气疗法

(1) 患者仰卧位。先按揉天枢、阑尾穴、足三里、上巨墟以通气机。再以平掌式按于脐部及阑尾点处用震颤手法（细微震颤）发气 28 息。

(2) 用平掌式以推拉手法，离开腹部向阑尾点处发气 14 息。并用拉引手法驱邪气外出。再用以上手法自腹部顺足阳明胃经向下肢导气 3 次或 7 次。

(3) 患者俯卧位，先按揉脾俞、胃俞、大肠俞。再以平掌式，用推拉颤手法顺足太阳膀胱经向下肢导气 3 次或 7 次。使上下气机平衡。

5.6 胆道疾患

胆道疾患主要有胆囊炎、胆石症和胆道蛔虫症等。祖国医学认为前者属于"胁痛"、"黄疸"等范围，而胆道蛔虫症则称为"蛔厥"或谓"虫心痛"。多因情志不舒，过食肥腻，或外邪侵袭。湿热蕴结，或虫积瘀阻，或驱蛔不当，蛔虫逆上，引起胆气郁结，疏泄失常所致。三者虽病因不同、症状少异，而气功锻炼和外气治疗方法基本一致，故合并叙述。

症状：本病发病较急，右上腹及右季胁部疼痛。常伴有恶心、呕吐、寒战、高烧，或见皮肤及巩膜黄染；若胆管完全梗阻，则可见灰白色粪便。深呼吸时胆囊有明显触痛。如系胆道蛔虫，剑突下剧烈绞痛，或呈钻顶撕裂样感觉。病人疼痛难忍，冷汗淋漓，可伴有恶心、呕吐。若蛔虫退出胆道，则疼痛可突然缓解，但可再度发作，若蛔虫体全部进入胆囊，则疼痛多呈持续性胀痛，也可出现黄疸、寒战、高烧等症状，剑突下偏右方有深压痛。

治疗：

1. 练功自疗

(1) 患者坐位或卧位，先练放松功，重点放松背腰部及胸腹部，反复放松。

(2) 练理肝功之摩胸嘘气法及疏肝导气法。

(3) 练胸胁功及腹部功。

2. 外气疗法

(1) 患者坐位。首先按揉脾俞、胃俞、肝俞、胆俞、胆囊穴（阳陵泉下2寸找压痛点）、足三里，均以右侧为主。

(2) 用平掌式，以震颤手法在右侧脾俞、胃俞及肝俞、胆俞处发气各28息。再在前侧疼痛处发气28息。

(3) 以平掌式、用拉颤手法在患者前侧胆区发气24息，并用拉引手法顺胆经、胃经向下导引气机，以疏泄胆气，宽中和胃。

(4) 按压右侧胆俞12息，并以按揉法在背腰部两侧膀胱经，自上而下，疏导气机3遍。

5.7 呃逆

呃逆俗称"打呃忒",是膈肌痉挛所致。常因过食生冷,嗜食辛辣或情志不畅,肝气犯胃,胃气上逆而致喉间呃呃连声。

症状:呃忒连声,轻者不经治疗持续数分钟或数小时可自愈,严重的可昼夜不停,以致影响进食、睡眠,致使病人疲惫不堪。如久病、重症突然并发此症,则多属危象,应加注意。

治疗:

1. 练功自疗

(1) 患者坐位或站位,面南背北,两脚与肩同宽,全身放松。以逆腹式呼吸,深吸一口气,呼气时以意引气下沉丹田,转而至两足拇趾之大敦穴处3息或9息。

(2) 练胸胁功及理肝功之摩胸嘘气法。

2. 外气疗法

(1) 患者坐位或站位,面南背北,全身放松,自然呼吸。医者先掐患者两中膈穴(中指屈曲,于第一指间关节拇指侧纹头尽处是穴),按揉脾俞、膈俞、膻中、中府、云门穴等。

(2) 以平掌式,用推拉引手法,向膻中发气,并顺足阳明胃经向两下肢导引,使气机调顺;再向背部脾俞、胃俞、肝俞发气,并顺足太阳膀胱经向下导气,使气机调顺。

(3) 症状仍不减轻者,再以平掌式,用推拉引手法向百会发气,并顺任脉向丹田导气,以引气归原。

5.8 胃下垂

胃下垂是一种慢性病,是指胃下降至正常位置以下而言。由于长期消化机能衰减,全身机能低下,营养不足,身体虚弱而致。中医学认为脾胃虚弱,中气下陷所致。

症状：本病以上腹部胀胞或腹胀，食后站立及举物时加重，卧位减轻为特点。伴有嗳气，泛酸或呕吐，纳食减少，消瘦，胃肠钡餐透视可确定诊断。

治疗：

1. 练功自疗

（1）练强壮功，以高尾姿势练功（仰卧位骶部垫高4寸），用逆腹式呼吸法。

（2）练延年九转功及腹部功。

2. 外气疗法

（1）患者取仰卧。先按中脘、提胃（脐上4寸）、胃上（脐上2寸旁开4寸）、足三里。

（2）用中指独立式，以震颤手法在中脘、胃上、提胃穴发气各14息；然后以平掌式，用震颤手法按在胃脘部发气14息。患者吸气有意，呼气无意。

（3）用平掌式，以推引手法向丹田发气14息，然后导气向胃府，再发气14息。

（4）按揉脾俞、胃俞，并以平掌式，用震颤手法向脾俞、胃俞发气14息，再以推引手法将膀胱经气机调顺。

5.9 泄泻

凡排便次数增多，粪便稀薄，甚至如水样，但无便血及里急后重者叫泄泻。多因内伤于饮食，或外感不正之气，以致胃肠不和，尤其夏秋之间，湿热盛行，暴注水湿者居多。更有脾肾阳虚而泄泻的慢性疾患，所谓肾虚则失其闭藏，脾虚则失其健运。此属内在的主要因素。

症状：本症依其发作原因和征象可分为三种：寒泻者肠鸣腹痛，大便泄泻，完谷不化，或如鸭溏，溲清不渴，脉沉迟，由于脾虚感寒者为多；热泻者泄泻黄糜气秽，肛门灼热，口渴烦躁，小便短赤，舌苔发黄，脉弦数，常有发热现象。由于感受暑热者多，五更泻者由于肾阳衰微，不能蒸化水谷，故又名肾泻。每在五更天将明时间泻 2～3 次。

治疗：

1. 练功自疗

（1）练周天自转功，只练自左向右转（逆时针方向），配合腹部功。

（2）受寒湿邪气者练涤秽功，五更泻者配合练采日精功。

2. 外气疗法

（1）先点按脾俞、胃俞、大肠俞，以开其俞穴；再以右手中指按其阑门穴，左手中指按鸠尾穴，开通此处之气机。

（2）用平掌式，以震颤手法在中脘、天枢、肚脐及关元穴各发功 14 息，摩腹 36 次（虚补实泻）。

（3）用平掌式，以推拉引手法施于腹部，导气或左或右旋转，并顺胃经向下导引。

（4）用平掌自龟尾推至第七胸椎。并按揉两侧膀胱经，按揉足三里。

（5）五更泻者以平掌式，用推旋手法向命门及丹田发气 9 息或 10 息。若寒湿泻或湿热泻者，当以平掌式，用拉引手法顺胃经向下导引，使气从足三里或解溪、足趾部排出。

5.10 便秘

便秘或独见或并发他病，推求其成因，有虚、实、风、冷、气、热之别。虚者是下焦阳虚或阴虚，如阳虚，则阴凝于下，无力运行。阴虚则津液失调，肠内干枯；实者胃实而秘；风者其人素有风疾，风盛则干；冷者，阴凝固结，气机闭塞；气者，气滞不行；热者，热灼津液。凡此种种，皆能促使便秘。

症状：

大便秘结不通，排便时间延长、或虽有便意而排出时甚为困难。有三、五日或六、七日左右大便一次者。虚冷者，此人少气，小便清白，大便实而难出；实热者喜冷食，小便赤；风冷者，喘咳气逆，形寒肢冷，大便难而腹痞满；气滞者，其人多噫，心腹痞闷，胸胁膜胀。

治疗

1. 练功自疗

(1) 练周天自转功，以顺时针方向运转为主，配合练腹部功，延年九转功。

(2) 属实热者，再练理脾功之摩脘呼气法。症属虚寒者，兼练理脾功之摩脘呼气法。

2. 外气疗法

(1) 按揉大肠俞、肾俞、八髎，以开其俞穴，再推下七节骨50次。

(2) 以两手拇指和中指开阑门穴，以通为度。再以平掌式，用震颤手法在中脘穴发气14息，然后以龙衔式，用推旋手法在天枢发气14息；并向关元发气8息，再向顺时针方向导引气机运行。

(3) 以平掌式，用推拉旋手法离开治疗部位发气8息。然后向顺时针方向导气，使气机活跃。

5.11 胁痛

《内经》云："邪在肝则两胁下痛。"这证明胁痛的原因，虽然有气滞、瘀阻、痰浊以及体质之或虚或实等不同，但无不与肝有关，尤其是肝阳素旺或肝气抑郁者，易见此症。

症状：胁肋疼痛，有一侧痛者，也有两侧痛者，而一侧者为多。实症者，痛势剧烈，甚则咳嗽，呼吸不利。若由肝实火盛者，两胁下痛，脉弦口苦；虚症者，如肝肾阴亏，或情志抑郁，或失血后所致者，则脉常柔弱，或咽喉干燥，或胃纳不甘，发作时其痛隐隐或刺痛。

治疗：

1. 练功自疗

（1）实症者，练理肝功之摩胁嘘字诀；虚症者，练理肾功之服黑气法，均配合练胸胁功。

（2）练延年九转功。

2. 外气疗法

（1）点按揉膻中、期门、章门、肝俞、膈俞、支沟、阳陵泉诸穴，以开其穴，疏通肝经之气血。

（2）以平掌式，用推拉引手法，向疼痛部位发功 11 息或 22 息。用拉引法，顺肝经向下导引气机。若两侧气机不平衡则左右导之。

（3）肝肾阴亏者，点关元、揉肾俞。再以平掌式，用颤法在小腹部，以关元为中心发功 8 息或 16 息。

5.12　支气管炎

本病是以咳嗽为主症的呼吸道疾患。急性支气管炎是由细菌、病毒感染或长期吸烟刺激所引起，慢性的多由急性支气管炎反复发作而致或继发于其他疾病。祖国医学认为本病属于咳嗽、咳喘、痰饮之类，多因风寒、风热之邪或痰湿内盛而致。

症状：急性支气管炎多属外感咳嗽。发病急，先有鼻塞、喉痒、干咳等上呼吸道症状，可伴有怕冷、发热、头痛和全身不适。咳嗽呈阵发性，可咳出稀痰或粘痰，苔薄白，脉浮紧。如风寒化热，则舌苔转黄，痰粘稠或呈脓性，脉多浮数或滑数。慢性支气管炎多属内伤咳嗽，常反复发作，秋冬两季或气候变化时易发病，清晨和傍晚咳嗽加重，痰量较多，苔滑腻，脉滑者属于痰湿内盛，如脓痰量多或痰中带血，脉细数，则为热伤肺络。若经年不愈，反复发作，可引起肺气肿。

治疗：

1. 练功自疗

(1) 虚症练理肺功中之服白气法；实症练理肺功之摩胸叫气法。均配合练理肺功之理肺导气法及胸胁功。

(2) 急性支气管炎有头痛、怕冷等表症者，练鼻齿功、头面功。

(3) 慢性支气管炎属脾肺气虚者，配合练理脾功之服黄气法。肾气不足者，练理肾功之服黑气法。均配合练强壮功。

2. 外气疗法

(1) 患者取坐位。先按揉膻中、肺俞，外感者加开天门，推坎宫，运太阳，按揉风门。

(2) 然后用平掌式，以推拉颤手法向膻中、肺俞发气各6息或12息。并顺肺经导引经气。

用震颤手法向中脘发气14息；再用平掌式，以推引手法顺胃经向下导引经气。

(3) 肺脾气虚者，用平掌式，以推拉手法向中脘、气海发气8息，并顺任脉导引经气，使气归原。肾气虚者，以平掌式，用推拉颤手法向丹田、命门发气各8息。

(4) 若外感风寒，邪气盛者，以平掌式，用拉引手法向膻中发气，并顺肺经导引邪气从指端出。

5.13 支气管哮喘

支气管哮喘是一种变态反应性疾病。多反复发作，呈阵发性而带哮鸣音的呼吸困难为主症。祖国医学认为每因感受风寒、饮食不节、情志抑郁、劳倦以致脾肺两虚，痰湿阻肺，肺失宣降，或下元不固，肾失摄纳而致。

症状：本病可分虚、实两种。实喘发病急剧，呼吸困难，张口抬肩，不能平卧，胸膈满闷，喉中痰鸣，脉浮紧，苔薄白。虚喘者则气短而促，动则喘甚，面色灰暗，汗出肢冷，舌质淡红，脉细弱无力。

治疗：
1. 练功自疗
(1) 选练放松功、内养功及胸胁功。
(2) 实症痰湿壅阻者，加理肺功之摩胸咽气法。脾肺气虚者，加练理肺功之服白气法和理脾功之服黄气法。肾不纳气，气短汗出者，加练理肾功之服黑气法。
(3) 可配合练铁裆功，用以益肾壮阳，增补元气。
2. 外气疗法
(1) 首先点揉定喘穴（大椎穴旁开0.5寸）及天突、膻中、关元、肺俞、脾俞、肾俞等穴。
(2) 以平掌式，用震颤手法在定喘、肺俞、脾俞发功各14息或28息。然后手式离开体表，以推拉引手法逆督脉向下导气至命门处。反复3~7次。
(3) 用龙衔式或平掌式，以推拉颤引手法发气于天突、膻中，然后顺任脉向丹田导气，使逆上之气下降。
(4) 肾虚，元阳不足者，用平掌式，以推拉手法发气于命门、肾俞、丹田，以壮肾之元阳。脾湿痰阻者，按揉丰隆，并用拉引手法发气于膻中，再导气于足阳明胃经，使痰湿之气顺胃经从足三里排出。

5.14 心悸

心悸是一种自觉心脏搏动异常的症状。常见于神经官能症及各种心脏病，祖国医学认为本病可因受惊恐或因心气、心血不足，心失所养而致心神不宁。

症状：自觉心慌、心跳不宁，可伴有胸闷、恶心呕吐等症多呈阵发性发作，常因情绪波动、劳累过度及过量饮酒或吸烟而发。

治疗：

1. 练功自疗

(1) 选练强壮功、内养功、胸胁功。

(2) 实症者练理心功之摩胸呵气法及理心导气法，虚症者练理心功之服赤气法及理心导气法。配合延年九转法。肾气不足者，配合练理肾功之壮肾导气法。

2. 外气疗法

(1) 先按揉心俞、肝俞、膻中、鸠尾、阑门，以开其穴，通其气机。

(2) 以中指独立式或剑诀式，用震颤手法发气于心俞、肝俞、膻中诸穴各8息；然后导引气机收归丹田。

(3) 惊恐或神志不宁者，以龙衔式，用震颤手法发气于睛明、印堂、百会各8息；然后离开穴位发气，用拉引法引气下行，使气机上下调顺。

5.15 遗精

遗精有梦遗与滑精两种。梦而遗精者，多因相火过旺，而阴精走泄，或心阳暗炽，肾阴内烁，或烦劳过度，心肾不交而导致。滑精者，无梦而遗、多由肾关不固，精窍滑脱。

症状：梦遗者，在睡眠中有梦而遗，或五、六天一次，或三、四天一次，伴有头昏眩晕，全身疲乏，腹部疼痛等。滑精者，无梦而泄，或动念即遗，不拘昼夜，四肢无力，记忆减退，甚者经年不愈。

治疗：

1、练功自疗

(1) 练倒阳功或回精还液功。配合练腰部功、理肾功等。

(2) 练养肾回春功及倒阳功。亦可选练铁裆功。

2. 外气疗法

(1) 按揉肾俞、心俞、命门、关元、中极、三阴交等穴。

(2) 以平掌式、用震颤手法发气于中脘、关元、命门各 8 息或 12 息。以平掌式，用推拉颤手法向丹田、命门发气，并顺督脉向上引至百会；然后转向前顺任脉引气归丹田。

(3) 以平掌式，用推引手法向百会发气 8 息。并顺任脉引归丹田。

5.16 阳痿

阳痿是阴茎痿而不举、或举而不坚的一种疾病。本病多由于青年犯手淫，或房事过度而致。其他如思虑劳精，或隐曲不遂，或惊恐伤肾，亦可导致本病。

症状：

阴茎不能健举，或举而不坚，随即萎缩，或兼见腰酸腿软。头昏目眩，精神萎靡，四肢乏力，记忆力减退等症。

治疗：

1. 练功自疗

(1) 首选铁裆功坚持锻炼，配合练习养肾回春功及腰部功。

(2) 肾气不足者，加练理肾功；身体衰弱，四肢乏力者，加练延年九转法、内养功或强壮功。精神萎靡不振者，练头面功。

2. 外气疗法

(1) 按揉肾俞、命门、关元、三阴交穴。

(2) 以平掌式，用震颤手法在关元穴发气 12 息；再以中指独立式，用震颤手法在中极穴发气 12 息；然后以平掌式，用推拉手法向命门穴发气 24 息。

(3) 以平掌式，用推拉旋引手法向命门、丹田穴发气 24 息，并左旋导气。

5.17 痛经

本病是在月经期以下腹部疼痛为主症的疾病。经常与经期情绪紧张，受寒饮冷有关。祖国医学认为受寒饮冷、忧思忿怒，情志郁结，气虚血少，皆可导致本病。痛经有虚实之分。

症状：实痛者，临经期前少腹痛或经常少腹痛，内热甚而口干燥，血色紫黑，多先期而经至，脉象多见弦数。虚痛者，每在经期后少腹痛，温热与手按即缓解，血色淡少，多过期行经，经常畏冷，脉象多见细滑。

治疗：

1. 练功自疗

(1) 练养肾回春功，配合练腹部功与腰部功。

(2) 加练周天自转功，实症者以顺时针方向转为主，虚症者以逆时针方向转为主。

(3) 身体虚弱者加练强壮功或内养功。

2. 外气疗法

(1) 先点揉气海、关元、中脘、肾俞，以开其穴。

(2) 以平掌式或中指独立式，用震颤手法发气于中脘、气海、关元。再以摩法旋摩小腹部，虚则补之，实则泻之。然后按揉三阴交、阴陵泉、太溪等穴。

(3) 以平掌式，用推拉旋手法向下丹田发气，并导气以脐为中心旋转，虚症右旋，实症左旋。

(4) 以平掌式，用定颤手法发气于命门、肾俞及骶部；再以引法导气顺膀胱经下行，使气机调顺。

5.18 慢性盆腔炎

慢性盆腔炎是指子宫、卵巢、输卵管、盆腔结缔组织等慢性炎症而言，多发于中年妇女。祖国医学认为由湿热或寒湿留滞胞宫所致。

症状：小腹疼痛、坠胀、腰骶酸楚、疼痛，每于经期或劳累后加重。阴道分泌物增多而成带下。急性期多伴有头痛、发热、恶寒等全身症状。如湿热者，带下多黄赤而有臭味，脉多滑数，舌苔黄腻。寒湿者，带下色白而腥臭，舌苔白腻，脉象沉迟或弦滑。

治疗：

1. 练功自疗

(1) 练强壮功、周天自转功、腹部功。

(2) 寒湿、湿热盛者，以化湿清热为主，加练涤秽功，理脾功之摩腹呼气法、理脾导引法。腰痛不适者加练腰部功。

2. 外气疗法

(1) 按揉中脘、带脉、中极、脾俞、命门、肾俞、三阴交诸穴。

(2) 以中指独立式，用震颤手法发气于中脘、气海、中极各8息。然后以平掌式、用推拉引手法发气于丹田、气海、中极、天枢；最后顺胃经向下导引，至气机平衡为止。

(3) 以平掌式，用推拉颤手法向命门、肾俞发气8息。然后理顺带脉，调左右之气脉，使其平衡为止。

5.19 子宫脱垂

子宫脱垂是指子宫位置下移至坐骨棘水平以下，或脱出于阴道口以外而言。如生育过多，产后失调或因他病，使子宫韧带松弛，当腹压增加，子宫被挤压而下垂。祖国医学称为"阴挺"，认为是由带脉失约，中气下陷，冲任不固或湿热下注所致。

症状：自觉阴部有物下垂，伴有腰酸，下腹部重坠感。严重者宫颈或子宫体全部脱出阴道口外，一般平卧时可上缩，起立行走可下垂。

治疗：

1. 练功自疗

(1) 采用仰卧高尾式姿势练内养功。配合练腹部功、腰部功（不练其中下推的手法）。

(2) 练周天自转功、理脾功之服黄气法。配合练通任督导引功或升降阴阳导引功。练功时重升轻降。

2. 外气疗法

(1) 按揉百会、气海、归来、脾俞、肾俞诸穴。

(2) 以平掌式或中指独立式，用震颤手法发气于百会、气海各8息，发气于脾俞、肾俞各14息。

(3) 用平掌式、以推拉颤手法发气于百会、命门、脾俞、肾俞、气海，并导引气机至中丹田，使气上升。

(4) 以平掌式，用推引手法发气于三阴交，并导气上行至中丹田，调顺气机。

5.20 乳痈

乳痈又叫吹乳，现代医学称为"乳腺炎"。多由肝胆之气郁结，胃经热毒壅滞，以致气血阻遏而发生乳痈。也有因乳部外伤挤压而引起乳汁壅滞而成者。乳儿口气不洁感染而致乳部发生炎症而肿痛者，名为吹乳。多见于女子哺乳期。

症状：初起乳房红肿、灼热疼痛，或结块如桃李，伴有寒热、恶心、烦渴等现象，继而局部成脓。

治疗：

1. 练功自疗

(1) 初起未成脓者，以食、中、无名、小指四指并拢，轻揉肿痛之周围。并练胸胁功。

(2) 练理肝功中之摩胸嘘气法与理脾功之摩腹呼气法。

2. 外气疗法：外气治疗宜初期尚未化脓之时，若已形成脓肿，应切开引流。

(1) 按揉膻中、乳根、中府、肝俞、胃俞以开通肝、胃、肺经之穴窍。

(2) 以平掌式，用震颤手法将内劳宫对准肿块发气 48 息。再用龙衔式，运气于指间，以震颤法发气 24 息。最后以平掌式，用推拉引手法发气于乳中穴并顺胃经下导经气、疏通经络，引胃气下行，驱邪气外出。

(3) 以拇、食、中三指在乳头后方轻轻捏挤，排出瘀积之乳汁。每天治疗一次。

5.21 落枕

落枕是指急性单纯性颈项僵痛、活动障碍的一种病症。多因睡眠姿式不当，或感受风湿邪气，经络失于通畅所致。

症状：一般多在早晨起床后一侧项部疼痛，转动不灵，疼痛可扩散至肩背部，肌肉呈痉挛状态和有明显的局部压痛，但无红肿发热。

治疗：

1. 练功自疗

练颈项功、肩臂功、配合练六段锦。

2. 外气疗法

(1) 先按揉天柱及颈部两侧膀胱经；再按揉风池、风府、肩中俞、肩外俞、曲池、合谷等穴，使经脉疏通，穴位打开。

(2) 用平掌式，以推拉引手法发气于颈部疼痛处，然后顺膀胱经向下导引，并顺小肠经向上肢导引，以疏通经络，调理气机。

(3) 用颈部斜板法以滑利关节、调理筋脉。

5.22 腰腿痛

腰腿痛多由于外感风寒或坐卧湿地，风湿袭入经络，或劳损，肾气虚弱，精气不足，或外伤所引起。相当于现代医学中腰椎间盘突出症、坐骨神经痛等症。

症状：属风寒湿者，腰部酸痛，不能俯仰转侧，甚则痛势延至腿足，每遇天阴加重，局部常有自觉寒冷感。肾虚腰痛者，隐隐而痛绵延不已，腰腿酸软无力，精神萎顿，脉象数而细。外伤腰腿痛者，腰部疼痛，压痛明显，或轻度肿胀，也可沿足少阳胆经或足太阳膀胱经向下肢放射性疼痛。

治疗：

1. 练功自疗

(1) 练腰部功及下肢功为主。

(2) 症状减轻后可练六段锦、易筋经能促使恢复及预防其复发。

2. 外气疗法

(1) 按揉肾俞、命门、腰阳关、环跳、阳陵泉、委中、承山、昆仑、太溪诸穴、以疏通经气。

(2) 以平掌式，用推拉引手法向命门、肾俞发气，并顺足太阳膀胱经向下肢导引。

(3) 以平掌式，用推拉引手法向环跳发气，并顺足少阳胆经向下肢导气，使经气平衡。

(4) 用腰部斜扳法，拍打法及腰、髋、膝部被动活动，以滑利关节，舒筋活血。

5.23 头痛

头痛是一种自觉症状，可出现于多种急慢性疾病中。祖国医学认为内伤、外感均可导致本病。如外感风寒，侵于头顶，随经入脑，或胃有积热，循经上逆，或气虚血亏，髓海失养，或痰湿内阻，清阳不升，或肝胆火旺等均可发头痛。盖头为诸阳之首，脏腑经络之气皆上会于头，故常以经脉循行部位而定头痛之名。

症状：

(1) 阳明头痛（前头痛）：阳明之脉循发际达额颅，故以前额痛为特征，伴有烦热燥渴，口臭便秘，舌苔黄，脉洪大有力或滑数。

(2) 少阳头痛（偏头痛）：少阳经脉行于头侧，故以偏侧头痛为其主症，头中炽热、疼痛如劈，或伴有目赤、胁痛、口苦、咽干、舌苔黄燥、脉弦数。

(3) 太阳头痛（枕后痛）：枕后项背为太阳之分野，故以枕后痛为其主症。可伴有发热、恶寒、项背僵痛、苔薄白，脉浮紧。

(4) 厥阴头痛（头顶痛）：足厥阴经脉会于头顶，故以头顶痛为主症，可兼见目眩、心烦易怒、面赤、口苦、失眠、舌红苔黄，脉弦数或细数。

治疗：

1. 练功自疗

(1) 练放松功，重点放松与疼痛有关经络的部分。如阳明头痛重点放松足阳明胃经与手阳明大肠经；少阳头痛主要放松足少阳胆经与手少阳三焦经；太阳头痛主要放松足太阳膀胱经及手太阳小肠经；厥阴头痛主要放松足厥阴肝经。

(2) 练头面功、延年九转功、六段锦功等。

2. 外气疗法

(1) 先据头痛的部位，按揉以下穴位：阳明头痛按揉印堂、头维、合谷、足三里；少阳头痛按揉太阳、悬颅、阳陵泉；太阳头痛按揉风府、风池、天柱、肩中俞、肩外俞、后溪；厥阴头痛按揉百会、阳陵泉、太溪。

(2) 以平掌式，用推拉引手法发气于疼痛部位；再用推引手法顺经自头部向下导引，使气下行。如侧头痛，先向疼痛侧发气，待气机明显后，用拉导手法顺手少阳三焦经向指端导引；然后顺足少阳胆经向下肢导引，以达气机下实上虚或平衡为原则。

(3) 再用平掌式，以推拉旋手法，调整左右前后，使其气机平衡。

5.24 失眠

本病以夜不能入眠为主症。祖国医学认为每因思虑过度，伤及心脾或精血耗损，或饮食不节，肠胃受损，皆可导致本病。

症状：以夜不得眠或难以入睡，或睡而易醒，难以再眠为主症。若伴有心悸、多梦、易醒、虚烦不眠、善惊易恐、或有盗汗、舌边尖红、脉弦细者，为心虚胆怯。若心悸健忘、神疲体倦、饮食无味、面色少华、舌淡苔薄、脉象细弱者，为心脾两虚。若兼见头晕健忘、耳鸣心悸、腰膝酸软、梦遗、舌质红少苔、脉象细数者，为心肾不交。若兼见脘腹胀满、嗳气、恶心、难以入睡，或大便不爽、苔淡黄而腻、脉沉而滑数者，为脾胃不和。

治疗：

1. 练功自疗

(1) 练放松功，配合练头面功。

(2) 心虚胆怯者，加练理心功。心脾两虚者，加练理心功、理脾功。心肾不交者练升降阴阳功或理心功、理肾功。脾胃不和者练理脾功、周天自转功。

2. 外气疗法

(1) 点按揉大椎、百会、太阳，推揉颔颜、率谷，点揉肝俞、肾俞、关元、气海，开其穴位，疏通经脉。

(2) 以平掌式，用震法发气于百会、大椎各 8 息或 16 息；发气于中脘、关元各 8 息或 16 息。然后用平掌式，以推引手法离开穴位向百会发气，并顺肾经引气向两涌泉穴，患者意守涌泉。

(3) 重复点揉百会、太阳，推颔颜、率谷等穴位，最后用击法于百会及大椎，摇两上肢。

(4) 心虚胆怯者，加用中指独立式，以震颤手法发气于心俞、肝俞、巨阙各 14 息；并用平掌式，以推引手法导引心经及胆经之气机，使其上下左右平衡。心肾不交者，加以中指独立式，用震颤手法发气于肾俞、心俞各 14 息；再用平掌式、以推引手法导引心经、肾经气脉，使其平衡。心脾两虚者，加用中指独立式，以震颤手法发气于脾俞、心俞各 14 息；并用平掌式，以推引手法顺脾经导引气脉，使其平衡。脾胃不和者，加用中指独立式，以震颤手法发气于脾俞、胃俞各 14 息；再用平掌式，以推引手法顺胃经导引经气，使其经气平衡。

5.25 高血压病

本病是指在安静休息时，如血压经常超过 18.7／12 千帕（140／90 毫米汞柱）即称为高血压。祖国医学认为本病是由于肝肾失调、阴阳偏盛或痰湿上扰所致。

症状：头痛、头胀、面红目赤、口干、心烦易怒、便秘、苔黄、脉弦数有力者，为肝火上炎；眩晕耳鸣，腰酸腿软，心悸失眠，舌质红绛，脉弦细而数者，为肝肾阴虚。如兼夹痰湿，则可见胸闷、肢麻、形盛肢胖，脉弦滑等。

治疗：

1. 练功自疗

(1) 练放松功，兼练头面功、颈项功、上肢功、下肢功。

(2) 肝火上炎者兼练理肝功之摩胁嘘气功，肝肾阴虚者兼练理肾功与理肝功。

2. 外气疗法

(1) 按揉阑门、中脘、关元，推天门、坎宫、太阳，点揉脾俞、胃俞、肝俞、胆俞、足三里，揉两侧膀胱经。

(2) 用平掌式，以震颤手法发气于百会、大椎、命门、中脘、关元各8息或16息；用中指独立式，以震颤手法发气于中脘8息；然后用平掌式，以推拉颤引手法离开治疗部位向百会、丹田发气。然后用推拉引手法顺胃经向下肢导引经气，使气机下实上虚。并用同法顺手阳明大肠经向肢端导引气机，使其平衡为止。

(3) 肝火上炎者，用平掌式，以推拉旋手法向肝俞、肾俞、丹田发气，并顺行旋转导引，以滋阴潜阳。肝肾阴虚者，用平掌式，以震颤手法在肾俞、丹田发气，滋肝肾之阴。

5.26 颈椎病

颈椎病又称颈椎退行性脊椎病，是40岁以上中老年人的一种常见病。祖国医学认为是由感受风寒湿邪、外伤，劳累，年老气血不足，血不养筋而造成的。

症状：颈椎病在临床上症状较为复杂，其中以颈神经根刺激或压迫症状（如颈项、肩臂肩胛上背、上胸壁及上肢疼痛或麻痛）为常见。患者往往因颈部过劳或感受寒冷而诱发此病或使症状加剧。若脊髓受到刺激或压迫，可出现下肢麻木失灵、无力、行走不稳等。若椎动脉受刺激或压迫，可出现头晕、头昏等。

治疗：

1. 练功自疗

(1) 练颈项功、肩臂功、六段锦等。

(2) 若出现头晕、头昏应加练放松功、头面功、理肝功。若出现下肢不稳、无力，加练下肢功、升降阴阳功。

2. 外气疗法

(1) 按揉风池、风府、天柱、肩中俞、肩外俞、极泉、曲池、合谷、少海、小海等穴，以通其气血。

(2) 用平掌式，以震颤手法在大椎穴发气16息。再用平掌式，以推拉引手法向颈部及大椎发气，并顺手三阳经导气于指端。

(3) 再按揉以上诸穴，并用拍法、击法、摇法、搓法结束治疗。

5.27 半身不遂

半身不遂系由外感风邪侵袭或肝风内动引起的中风后遗症。

症状：口眼歪斜，半身不遂，舌僵语蹇，手足痿而不用等症。

治疗：

1. 练功自疗

(1) 加强患肢的活动。

(2) 以健肢握空拳拍打患肢，自上而下3~5遍。

(3) 以健肢拉患肢。吸气时向上内等方向牵拉，呼气时放松，并意想气达患肢。

(4) 练上肢功、下肢功、头面功等。

2. 外气疗法

(1) 按揉合谷、颊车、内关、曲池、阳陵泉、委中，掐指端及指甲两侧。

(2) 按揉背部膀胱经，自上至下6~7次。

(3) 以平掌式或剑诀式，用推拉引手法向印堂、百会发气，然后导气下行。

(4) 以平掌式，用推拉引手法向大椎、风门、肝俞、肾俞发气，并用同法自头之左侧经颈部向右侧导气；再自头之右侧经颈部向左侧导气，使气机平衡。

5.28　近视眼

近视眼多发于青少年，与看书时灯光照明不好、姿势不正、连续看书时间过长等有关。

症状：看远模糊，看近清楚。

治疗：

1. 练功自疗

练疏肝明目功、眼功等。

2. 外气疗法

(1) 按揉睛明、球后、印堂、太阳、风池、合谷、光明等穴。

(2) 用一指禅式或剑诀式，以推拉手法，或用中指独立式，以震颤手法，向睛明、肝俞、肾俞发气各14息。

(3) 用平掌式，以推拉引手法向眼部发气，并顺胆经导引，使气机平衡。

5.29　小儿惊症

小儿惊症多因小儿受惊吓而引起。

症状：小儿烦燥不安，或精神萎靡，夜啼不眠，厌食，腹泻或发热等症。

治疗：

1. 揉小天心，掐心经，掐肝经，掐五指节，掐印堂，掐百会。

2. 以平掌式，用推拉引手法向小儿囟门、百会处发气，并顺任脉向丹田导气，引气归原。

3. 再用平掌式，以推拉引手法向大椎、心俞、肝俞发气，将膀胱经及督脉经气调顺。

5.30　小儿腹泻

小儿腹泻多因感受寒湿、暑热之邪气，或因内伤乳食，脾胃虚弱等。

症状：大便稀，次数多，消化不良。寒湿者大便清稀多沫，肠鸣腹痛；湿热者，腹痛即泻，暴注下迫、大便色黄热臭，发热口渴等；伤食者，腹痛腹满，泻后痛减，大便臭秽；脾虚者，久泻不愈，反复发作，每于食后泻等。

治疗：

1. 按揉脾俞、胃俞、大肠俞、天枢、中脘、丹田。

2. 以平掌式，用震颤手法向中脘、天枢、关元各发气 8 息或 16 息；再以平掌式，用推拉旋手法向腹部发气，并旋转导引，或补或泻相机行事。

3. 实热症者，用平掌式，以拉引手法向中脘发气，并导邪气外出。

4. 脾胃虚弱者，用平掌式，以推定手法向中脘、丹田发气，以补元气。

THE ENGLISH–CHINESE ENCYCLOPEDIA OF PRACTICAL TCM

(Booklist)
英汉实用中医药大全

(书目)

VOLUME	TITLE	书名
1	ESSENTIALS OF TRADITIONAL CHINESE MEDICINE	中医学基础
2	THE CHINESE MATERIA MEDICA	中药学
3	PHARMACOLOGY OF TRADITIONAL CHINESE MEDICAL FORMULAE	方剂学
4	SIMPLE AND PROVEN PRESCRIPTIONS	单验方
5	COMMONLY USED CHINESE PATENT MEDICINES	常用中成药
6	THERAPY OF ACUPUNCTURE AND MOXIBUSTION	针灸疗法
7	*TUINA* THERAPY	推拿疗法
8	MEDICAL *QIGONG*	医学气功
9	MAINTAINING YOUR HEALTH	自我保健
10	INTERNAL MEDICINE	内科学

11	SURGERY	外科学
12	GYNECOLOGY	妇科学
13	PEDIATRICS	儿科学
14	ORTHOPEDICS	骨伤科学
15	PROCTOLOGY	肛门直肠病学
16	DERMATOLOGY	皮肤病学
17	OPHTHALMOLOGY	眼科学
18	OTORHINOLARYNGOLOGY	耳鼻喉科学
19	EMERGENTOLOGY	急症学
20	NURSING	护理学
21	CLINICAL DIALOGUE	临床会话

The English—Chinese
Encyclopedia of Practical TCM
Chief Editor   Xu Xiangcai

8
MEDICAL QIGONG

English Chief Editor   Yu Wenping
Chinese Chief Editor Bi Yongsheng

英汉实用中医药大全
主编 徐象才

8
医学气功

中文   英文

主编 毕永升 于文平

*

高等教育出版社出版
高等教育出版社照排中心照排
新华书店总店北京科技发行所发行
国防工业出版社印刷厂印刷

*

开本 850×1168 1/32 印张 13.5 字数 340 000
1990年10月第1版 1990年10月第1次印刷
印数 0001—5 250
ISBN 7-04-002060-2/R·1
定价 3.50元